For Promise ~
May you know
your many gifts ~
In light and love ~
Eve

UNEXPECTED GIFTS

My Journey with
My Father's Dementia

EVE SOLDINGER

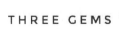

THREE GEMS PUBLISHING

Cover Design: Daniel Wolfsong

Author's Photo: Richard Rosenthal

Unexpected Gifts, by Eve Soldinger, is a powerful gift to anyone caring for a family member. While most books about dementia and caregiving focus on the losses experienced, Eve instead captures with beautiful clarity the pure distillation of the love she and her dad shared, and the gifts she experienced by being fully present with him. She opened her heart, and through her gentle but keen observations, helped to open the hearts of nearly everyone who came into contact with her beloved dad during the last years of his life. Every family member I have worked with who has had Eve's courage and grace to truly travel the journey of their loved one's last years, months, or days, has felt the blessings of the remarkable experience that she so beautifully articulates. *Unexpected Gifts* is a book to be treasured.

Susy Elder Murphy, Aging Life Care™ Manager

Unexpected Gifts is an astute portrait of the Soldinger family as they dealt with dementia. This stage of life is feared by many, on behalf of ourselves as well as our loved ones. Eve Soldinger shines a light on the love and growth that are still possible in this stage in life, individually and as a family. *Unexpected Gifts* is a must-have companion for every caregiver and should be on the reading list of physicians and other clinicians helping patients and their families navigate this road.

Dr. Charlotte Dean, Hospice and Palliative Care Physician

How does one thrive after a dementia diagnosis? Eve Soldinger paints a warm and affectionate portrait of her late father, Reuben Soldinger, whose descent into dementia challenges their love. With great tenderness, the writer weaves her tale of suffering with surprising threads of blessings. *Unexpected Gifts* is a gift to all of us who yearn for clarity in the midst of chaos.

Rabbi Tamara Miller, Washington, DC
www.RabbiTamaraMiller.com

Unexpected Gifts is an important book, a gem, that speaks clearly from the heart. Eve Soldinger bravely shared the trials of her undeniably difficult journey in great detail. The upsets were quickly and masterfully followed by deep questions that continue ringing and reverberating into the soul. Just when I felt my heart starting to swell, and expecting to break with the sadness of it all, Eve showed a path of lightheartedness. Reading it I was transformed. Eve gave me the gift of seeing both of my living parents in a more expansive light that I feel grateful to be experiencing now.

Roxanne Chan, OMD, Spring Wind Acupuncture, Anchorage, AK

It is said that the Torah's command "Honor your father and mother" is not so concerned with young children but with adult children and their aging parents. In *Unexpected Gifts*, Eve Soldinger honors her father with a moving meditation on the effects his dementia has on their loving relationship. Anyone affected by aging and dementia will be moved by the honor and love in this book. It is a gift!

Rabbi Edward C. Bernstein, Temple Torat Emet, Boynton Beach Florida; Editor, Love Finer Than Wine: The Writings of Matthew Eisenfeld and Sara Duke

In life we are given a series of challenges not of our choosing. In her moving memoir, Eve Soldinger provides us with an example of how finding the present moment and an open heart during traumatic times can lead to spiritual and emotional growth at any age. *Unexpected Gifts* is an inspirational account of self-realization and transformation.

Dr. Tony D'Angelo, DMQ, Tranquil Cloud Temple, Chicago, IL, Taoist Priest

DEDICATION

This book is dedicated to all who search for meaning as their loved ones suffer losses from dementia.

Preface

My dad, Reuben Soldinger, was ill for nearly two years. His mind was confused about many things. Sometimes he thought he was at a hotel, not in a nursing home. Often he didn't recognize my mother. Some days, he thought his son was his brother. But he was so much more than his forgetfulness. He was clever. He maintained a sense of humor. He still had a sense of amazement. He remained engaged in life.

His confusion defined his existence. He knew he was confused at least half of the time and wondered what he could do about it. He looked for the train, or he tried to do his job, or he gave a speech. But confusion was where he lived. He didn't know his age, the year, or his surroundings, but he did know that he could still have an impact on things. He knew it until his last days.

On this path he went forward with his heart. His mind no longer shielded him from feelings that he didn't want to face. Every emotion was authentic. There was truth in his interactions. Each moment was new, but it was also full of love, anger, or fear, and he had to travel through it.

Through this journey with my father I have been transformed. I walked the narrower path of being awake to the present moment. Before his illness, I had a very good relationship with my dad. Yes, it was laced with dramatic strife in my teenage years, miscommunications as adults, some disagreements and sometimes a lack of real understanding; but mostly he was my primary source of support and my loving guide for how to be in the world. Our relationship, as is true in most relationships, relied on past history for understanding each other. As this information became less available during his illness, I had the opportunity to see and hear him differently. The pain and the tragedy of it all was there, but so was the heart's ability to love, and the ability to see and hear his spirit, and this became the avenue for many unexpected gifts.

Dad changed. And he grew. Growing happens all throughout life, even at the end. I recognized his spiritual and emotional shifts and asked many questions along the way. How does one walk with someone who doesn't function within the social norms? How do I see to the needs of my beloved parent? And most important, how can I accompany him?

Accompanying Dad on this journey has been an honor. This writing is a tribute to who he was as a human being and a tribute to the growth that happens in every moment of life.

Thank you, Dad.

Chapter 54, Lau Tzu's Taoteching, Translated by Red Pine

What you plant well can't be uprooted

what you hold well can't be taken away

your descendants will worship this forever

cultivated in yourself virtue becomes real

cultivated in your family virtue grows

cultivated in your village virtue multiplies

cultivated in your state virtue abounds

cultivated in your world virtue is everywhere

thus view others through yourself

view families through your family

view villages through your village

view states through your state

view other worlds through your world

how do you know what other worlds are like

through this one

Chapter 1
Finding Dad

February 20, 2003.

My niece Laurie found Dad lying on the kitchen floor.

My father and mother lived in a large house in Orlando, with my brother, Craig, their primary caretaker. Craig had made a midmorning check-in call from work to our parents. No answer.

Mom, at 83, slept late into the mornings; it was normal that she wouldn't hear the call. But my father, despite his 89 years and an array of ailments befitting his age, would have been awake, perusing the paper and checking on the stock market. He looked at the ads and scanned the op-ed page. Each month he wrote me a letter in which he shared some of his opinions.

Craig called, again and again, for a half hour. Then he called Laurie, his daughter, who lived just two miles away from my parents. Laurie called for about 15 minutes before she decided to load her two 3-year-old daughters and 1-year-old son into the car. She checked the sidewalks as she drove, to see if my dad might be taking a walk, even though Craig had said Dad didn't take walks on his own anymore.

Laurie pulled the minivan into the garage, opened the doors, and told her children to stay in the car.

Stepping into the house, she called out: "Poppie? Bubbie?"

No answer.

She heard a noise from the direction of the kitchen. But she didn't see anyone.

One more time: "Bubbie? Poppie?" Then, from behind the kitchen counter, she clearly heard my dad say, "Is that you, Sally?"

Sally was my father's sister. Dad hadn't seen Sally for years. Sally lived in Arizona, being cared for near her daughter. Something was wrong.

Laurie walked behind the kitchen counter and found Dad on the floor, in his blue bathrobe and slippers. She saw blood on his knuckles and a cut on his head. Her first thought was that he shouldn't get up. He might have broken bones. Maybe his confusion meant he had had a stroke.

She called 911. Dad tried to talk, but he was mumbling, and she could no longer understand his words.

She placed a pillow under his head. "You're going to be okay. I'm here. An ambulance is coming."

Dad tried to prop himself up on his elbow. Laurie thought he looked embarrassed to have been found lying on the kitchen floor in his bathrobe and slippers. He positioned himself as comfortably as he could, as if to convince her that he was okay, or, she thought, to give the impression that he somehow intended to be there.

She called Craig, who left right away to come home. She couldn't reach her husband, Scott, so called her in-laws to take care of the children. She didn't want the children to be alarmed about what was happening to their Poppie Rube.

Laurie heard my mother snoring in the other room. Mom had always been a night owl and could be up until 4 a.m., often sleeping until noon the following day. Laurie decided not to wake her and have to deal with her possible panic—she was already divided in her attention between caring for Dad and for her children.

The EMTs arrived, bringing in equipment.

"Do you know your name?" one asked Dad.

"Yes," Dad said.

"What is it?"

"Reuben."

"Do you know what day it is?"

He hesitated.

"Do you know what season it is?"

"Spring."

"What city are we in?"

"Orlando," he replied.

"What happened?"

"Can't remember." He continued to try to talk, but it was mostly mumbling.

"Any medical conditions?"

"Yes," answered Laurie. "He's diabetic."

"Medications?"

"Yes, I'll go get them."

In the bedroom Laurie grabbed all of both Mom's and Dad's medications and began sorting through the bottles to find the ones with Dad's name.

Laurie's father-in-law arrived to get the children. They weren't troubled—just in awe of the siren and the men from the fire truck.

The EMTs told Laurie that Dad's vitals were okay, but his oxygen was low, so he needed to go to the hospital.

My brother arrived just as the ambulance was leaving. He woke my mom, who was groggy and upset.

At the hospital, Laurie saw that Dad couldn't sit still. He kept rubbing his head. She tried to help by reminding him to keep his arms at his sides. Meanwhile, Craig handled communications: calling me, in California, and my sister, Jan, in Maryland, while also talking to my mother and the doctors and trying to keep things calm for Dad.

Dad seemed aware and apologetic that he wasn't his normal self. He was having trouble speaking and responding.

I didn't talk with Dad that day. Between phone calls with my family, I thought back to my last visit to my parents, just three weeks before. Dad had been as he usually was—self-contained, consistent, kind, and humorous.

But during that visit, I did notice that he had become thinner. Family members in Orlando had warned me about his weight loss. Dad had been 5 feet 8 inches and 140 pounds. He was aware of his diet and maintained a steady weight. He was proud of his self-discipline. Now he had shrunken to my height—about 5 feet 6 inches—and had lost 20 pounds.

I noticed the weight loss as soon as I walked into their home. But what I remember most is that my parents were all smiles. There was spirit in both of them. At 9:30 p.m. Florida time, but 6:30 California time, I scrounged around the kitchen looking for something light for my dinner.

I made the obvious joke that it looked like Dad was the one who needed to eat. His piercing blue eyes twinkled as he responded, "Oh, I ate well. I'm doing my part. I'm even drinking Ensure."

I laughed, joining in with his good humor. "Well, if this is the effect, maybe I should be drinking Ensure to lose weight, and you should try my diet of veggies and rice. I'll gladly throw in my extra pounds."

My Dad and I often joked about making trades. I had inherited his curly hair, but the passing decades had left him with a crown of white curls around an otherwise bald head. He would ask whether I had a chunk of hair to spare.

I found some applesauce and made some toast, while sharing stories of my recent trip and what I was up to. Dad was an intense listener. I counted on that, and looked to him for advice. Although my life took unconventional paths—studying Traditional Chinese Medicine, being an acupuncturist, and exploring healing traditions—he was always supportive. For the past few years, I had told him about my frequent travels through Guatemala, meeting with Mayan Elders, and visiting ancient cities, and he would say that he would like to join me. I told him that we could always find a wheelchair for the hikes, if he meant it. He didn't really mean it.

◇

That last visit was really meaningful. Dad and I talked about my future, my goals, and what kind of life I wanted to create as I neared 50 years. I had been living in California for the past year and was still deciding whether it was a comfortable place for me. Should I move back east, to Florida—or listen to the call to move to Tucson? We went over the values that might influence my life in each place. Florida had an obvious draw: It was close to Dad, Mom, and Craig, as well as to Laurie and my great-nieces and great-nephew.

On my last day there, I woke at 4:30 a.m. for my early flight back to California. Everything was more or less packed. I just needed to make sure that I hadn't forgotten anything. I walked into the kitchen, and there was Dad in his PJs, blue robe, and bedroom slippers.

"Dad, you didn't have to get up."

"I am glad to. Are you all set for the trip? Do you want to take some food for the flight? How about this applesauce? We have some plastic spoons somewhere."

So I took the food and thanked him. He walked outside with me with a wistful look. It was a very familiar look. It said *I already miss you.* It was a pitch dark January morning, except for the streetlights. But it was easy to see his sadness as he said goodbye.

"Dad, I have more work here next month, so I'll see you then," I said. "I love you." I thought to myself how lucky I was to have him as a father. He was so kind and loving.

I flew back to California and settled into a new apartment, excited to find my own path and set new goals for an unknown future.

Then on Valentine's Day, as I had for every Valentine's Day since I was 18 years old, I received a heartfelt note from Dad:

Dear Eve,

It seems like everything in our lives is working in double time, even if our normal routines are dull. However, things are OK if you ignore the TV and newspapers. They have to ignore the people who read.

Today is a day to use your heart for those we love. We all love you.

Hope you have a full day and life of love.

We hope to see our twins and Dylan. They sure love you. They wonder about you – so far away. So happy they'll see you again soon.

I've run into some financial problems again—dental problems—have to replace an upper set—-$1200, so I'll have to wait awhile to send your additional money. But you'll get it eventually.

Hope good things happen to you.

Love you so much,

Dad

Happy Birthday, Happy Valentine's

Dad wrote letters. I counted on his thoughtful and encouraging words. I would often find his letters saved as bookmarks or in my purse, reminders to have faith in myself, in God, and in the future. I always knew that I had a dad who stood behind me no matter what course I decided to take, even if he didn't understand it. With this Valentine's Day letter, I felt the tug. A part of me wanted to fulfill his wish to live closer to the family, but not before I could feel what I wanted next for myself. I knew that I was in the middle of a process.

I called and thanked him for the card and the check, and to wish him and my mom the most loving Valentine's Day ever. That was

February 14, 2003.

Now, a little over a week after my father wrote his Valentine's letter, he could hardly form sentences. But an MRI did not show signs of a stroke. The doctors were starting to talk about dementia.

It surprised me. Had I noticed anything during my visit? He did refer to someone's daughter as his sister. But he laughed at himself when he made the mistake. I could have made that same kind of mistake.

But I did recall there had been one strange moment. The last night I was there, Dad gave me a flashlight before I went to bed, "just in case I needed it." That was a little unexpected. Why would I need a flashlight? I remember exchanging glances with my brother, wondering what Dad was thinking. But in truth, he was oriented to time and place and was no more forgetful than I was.

Over the three years before this, Dad had experienced two small strokes called Transient Ischemic Attacks, or TIAs. A TIA can leave a person confused, unable to speak, or with trouble moving. In Dad's case, each time, after a few confusing days, he had made a complete recovery. I hoped that this was what happened this time.

The hospital wanted to send him home, but he was still unsteady on his feet. Our family asked to talk with a social worker about what to do next. Her assessment, combined with the huge change we could see in Dad, led to our decision to bring him to a nursing home for rehabilitation. He might have to be there several weeks, we imagined, until he got his strength and abilities back.

I wasn't too worried, but it did change all my plans. I needed to go to Florida.

For years, I had been the designated caregiver in the family. Even before I went into health care, in the 1970s, if anyone was ill or in the hospital, I was the family member who did the caregiving. I always thought my sister Jan was as good as I was in being present and sympathetic and doing whatever was needed, but somehow it was my domain.

Three years earlier, after one of Dad's TIAs, I had gotten medical power of attorney for my parents, so that I could be helpful and have some authority for just these kinds of situations. But despite this kind of preparation, I hoped this wouldn't be needed and I just wanted my dad to return to "normal."

I called just before getting on the plane for Florida. *His speech is getting better,* I thought. But he could no longer handle long conversations. Normally, we talked for at least 10 minutes, but not that day.

So I left California, trying to focus on the now but entrenched in the past, hopeful that I would soon have my dad back for long conversations—guiding me, discussing personal and world events, and being my friend.

I didn't recognize then, as we often fail to realize at the time, that there had been a fundamental shift in Dad, in his health and in who he was. My last visit and his Valentine's letter remained the lasting memories of the way things had been.

Chapter 2
All the World's a Play

When I visited Dad for the first time in the nursing home, I found him sitting in a wheelchair. As I walked down the hall towards him, I could see his head bobbing up and down. I wondered if he was tired or drugged. Then suddenly, as if from a sleep, he woke and spotted me.

"Evie!" he said, a shocked expression on his face. I watched his expression quickly shift to relief, and quick tears came to his eyes. As he attempted to get up, an alarm went off. The alarm didn't seem to matter to him, but it signaled an aide to shoo Dad back into the chair. He grasped my hand in an unfamiliar, desperate way.

"I'm so glad to see you," he said.

Minutes after my arrival, he was called to participate in group physical therapy exercises. I went with him and watched from the doorway. Dad tried to be a good patient and lift his arms straight up as instructed by the therapist leading the group. He put much attention and effort into doing the exercises. Some of the other people hardly responded to the therapist and she had to coax them to move with the rest. After 15 minutes, the lesson was over, and aides arrived to help the residents return to their rooms.

I was clueless about nursing homes. This one looked beautiful, but I didn't know what to look for or what to expect. I also had no idea what constituted "getting better." What would that mean for Dad? How could we evaluate how he was doing?

As I wheeled Dad back to his room, he said: "You know, it would be a much better play if the Irish would just rehearse. But they won't do it." He shook his head, giving the impression of great disappointment. It was quite emotional for him.

I was shocked. What was he talking about? Dad had spent time in World War II in Ireland and held a love of all things Irish. But who were the Irish in that room? Were they all the residents at physical therapy? I had just gotten there, and I already saw our realities no longer matched. He was different in so many ways.

One striking difference was that I noticed Dad stealing kisses when a nurse's aide extended her arms across his body. Dad's head innocently lowered to the skin of her arm as if he was having a moment of sleepiness, and when he reached the arm he placed a kiss. He then looked up at the woman with a flirtatious smile. I turned my head and laughed, wondering whether an apology was in order. I didn't notice anyone else there stealing kisses.

Who was this man? He had never behaved inappropriately toward women. He had really good boundaries. A few years earlier, when Mom and Dad briefly tried assisted living, Dad complained that some of the single older women would suddenly pinch his buttocks. He was shocked, and tried to avoid them. When someone wasn't behaving appropriately, it was a shock to him. Dad had always had a rigid code of behavior. Stealing kisses wasn't a part of his repertoire.

Over the next few days, I spent as much time as I could with him. I ran for a nurse's aide if he wanted to go to the toilet, and ran to get him water, his slippers, or his eyeglasses, as needed. But mostly I tried to arrange my visits to coincide with meals.

This was familiar to us both. I have eaten more meals with Dad than with anyone else in my family. We were the two early birds in the family. We would meet in the kitchen, he with a coffee and bagel while I found some fruit or oatmeal. He read the paper and I read a book, and we would talk, listening to each other's opinions or complaints. Quiet was rare. Dad was interested in other people's lives, and especially in the lives of his family members.

But in the nursing home, our mealtimes together bore no similarity to our past experiences. He could hardly eat. I easily fell into the role of coaxing him to eat. He was not interested. I took the problem to someone at the nurse's desk, only to find out that according to their record keeping, he was eating 100 percent of his meals. This was impossible, I told the head nurse. If he couldn't eat at lunch, I couldn't imagine that he was ravenous at breakfast. Whatever was wrong with my father, it was becoming clear that there was a lack of care and attentiveness at this facility.

That day, I was fighting a cold, so I left to take care of myself. I had lain down for only an hour when I received a call that Dad's breathing was shallow—he was being sent to the nearest hospital.

After only a week at the nursing home, he was back in the hospital. The pace of constant change was confusing enough to me and my family. How much more confusing could it have been to Dad?

So here we were dealing with another hospital within a week's time.

I was still adjusting to his condition and wondering where my father went and who it was that had suddenly replaced him. The speed of both physical and mental changes was difficult to witness. I needed time to have my own reactions of fright and horror. Yet I had to be present to assess his current situation and think about what the long-term effects might be.

What we learned at the hospital was that Dad was dehydrated, and his blood sugar was very low. Dehydration is one of the most significant complaints in nursing home care. My father's diabetes had been complicated from his difficulty in eating. Given what I had seen, I wasn't too surprised. I had just begun to confront the health care workers about his needs and take action to work things out with the people there—but with this episode, I realized things were not going to work out at that nursing home.

Most states have an agency that evaluates the care given in nursing homes and rates the standard and quality of care. Checking with the state agency is one of the most important things that one can do to ensure that a loved one is receiving the best care available. It would have been better to check this before transferring Dad from the hospital to the nursing home, but we didn't know that at the time. It was such an overwhelming time with my father's changes and feeling the desire to be there to hold his hand. The situation required that we pay attention to the details and not surrender authority. My brother and sister and I were coming to realize that we now represented my father's interests.

At the hospital emergency room, a large crew of us waited—my mother, Craig, Jan, Laurie, her husband, Scott, and close friends of the family from Jacksonville. Our family's usual way of handling emergencies is to use humor, but we were all so sure that Dad's death was imminent that I can't remember a single joke. The emergency room personnel insisted only two people at a time could be with Dad.

Dad seemed gaunt and lost, despite trying to be engaged with us. He wanted to talk about a beautiful party that he was organizing, where everyone would dress beautifully and wear diamonds. We would be picked up by limousines, and eat by 9 p.m., and then there would be dancing by 10 p.m., and we would smoke beautiful cigarettes, he said.

He was awake and alert, but not in the present reality. The hospital personnel said an infection might explain the delirium, so they ran tests. They found he had a bladder infection. So this seemed like good news—something that could be treated.

But another shock followed when the ER doctor gave his assessment: It sounded as if my father was dying, and he didn't have very long, perhaps two months. For the time being, the doctor said, we needed to think about using a feeding tube.

Our family went into red alert. Dad was admitted to the hospital and we each left with an assigned research task. My niece looked for articles on feeding tubes. I left imperative messages with colleagues who worked as nurses, doctors, and social workers, asking for advice. It felt like we needed to make an immediate decision. Would we agree to do this to my father if the primary reason was to control the complications of diabetes?

We each struggled to cope with our initial adjustment to his huge mental and physical changes. How would we come together to make this decision? Dad had not been capable of making decisions for a few days now, but could we assume authority about what was best for him? Would we agree? And could I manage to release my own hope—and denial—that he would simply wake up better, tomorrow?

We held our very first family meeting the next morning. Though we tried not to be dramatic, we had to project what Dad would want, consider the limitations of the information available, and share what we might glean from articles and advice. Most everyone was against the feeding tube. My mother could only talk about love and how our communication in these difficult moments was a testament to our family. We all saw that she had nothing to say about the decisions we had to make. As she aged, she had become increasingly fragile, physically and emotionally. Before this, she was the person in the couple who required constant care. One of the reasons I had medical power of attorney was because of her increasing inability to take in any information and take action. Scott, my niece's husband, and I were the only ones who thought a temporary feeding tube would be okay. No one else agreed with us. We conceded to majority rule. As soon as the meeting ended, Jan, and I hurried to the hospital, in the hope of being there when the internist made his visit.

The night before, we had spent the entire evening in the ER, leaving the hospital only when we were certain Dad would be cared for properly while the family figured out what to do next. But when we arrived at his hospital room, I had yet another shock.

Dad cried out: "Eve, Jan! Oh, thank God." Each of his hands was tied to the hospital bed. He was beside himself with anxiety. He looked like he had been crying. We ran to his bedside.

Every part of me was enraged at seeing this gentle man tied up. "Jan, help me to undo these," I said.

She asked why they had done this. It was obvious to me. They couldn't control Dad. I'm sure that, with no one to sit with him, he kept getting up. The nurses had to make sure that he didn't hurt himself. He couldn't remember to use the nurse call button. How else do hospitals deal with patients with dementia?

People in this situation need sitters, but instead hospitals use restraints on our elders, people in their 80s and 90s. And a person already confused finds him or herself with no control at all—and no sense of why they are restrained.

Despite having at least three phone numbers for our family, the hospital did not call to ask us to come sit with him.

We realized Dad now needed one of us with him to run interference in ways he never had before. If not, as in this case, he might be tied to the bed and left unable to express his needs. Now, we could be with him, and use the nurse's button for him, when he needed anything. And we knew that someone had to be there with him all the time.

I was the one with Dad when a doctor checked in. I immediately shared the conversation our family had had that morning about the feeding tube. But this doctor didn't seem to think that a feeding tube was called for. He said Dad needed his medications for diabetes straightened out and he needed his appetite stimulated.

At these types of moments, I started to feel like a pinball. One doctor told us Dad was dying, while the other said that the primary problem was to manage the diabetes. We all responded on so many levels to what the doctor had said the night before, making our emotional adjustments and sorting through medical information. Now, this doctor thought that was irrelevant.

But as this doctor asked Dad a few questions, I observed how masterful my father truly was at human relationships.

The doctor asked: "Where do you live?"

Dad answered in his usual tone, quite sure of himself: "North America."

"Where in North America?"

"North."

"Are you in a hotel, hospital, or home?"

My father replied, with only a slight hesitation: "I live in a very comfortable living environment."

"Do you know why you are here?"

"Yes," my father said, nodding. And with great emphasis and a loud voice, Dad answered, "I'm almost 90 years old."

Despite my concern, I was amused. Dad was literally correct in all his answers. But it was clear that even his ability to read people, and maintain a conversation could not disguise that he was confused and was not oriented to time and place. He hadn't been like this last month. He had lost that sense of appropriateness that had been a given my entire life. I chuckled, thinking how many times I had described my dad being "socially acceptable" or "extraordinarily appropriate." Sometimes I also described him as a conservative human being, but a kind man and a liberal in politics. But his consistency was gone. What could I count on from him? Where were his consistency and reliability?

My father put his hands behind his head, and in a very measured fashion said to the doctor: "Doctor, I don't know you, or what your medical education was like, but I have some advice for you." The doctor gave his full attention.

Dad paused dramatically and said, "Doctor, you should take more vacations. Try taking a month at a time, while you are still young."

The doctor made a swift exit from the hospital room, not needing any further information or advice from my father.

I laughed from somewhere deep inside, wondering whether this had been an original thought from Dad. It sounded as if the advice was off the cuff and not really a thought, but more a declaration of his role as the advice-giving elder in this situation with this much younger man. Even if Dad was confused, he had mastered the art of claiming greater authority.

I excused myself from Dad and ran to catch up with the doctor on his way to the elevators to ask him what we might expect. His words loom large in my memory.

First, he told me that Dad's medical condition would improve, but his dementia would only get worse. And he asked whether we planned to take him home. I didn't know. How could we manage him? What would his needs be? I didn't recognize him already. Who was this man who, when his hospital roommate was wheeled back in from X-ray, shouted out heartily: "Hello, fellow traveler!" I liked much about this new man, but I missed the reliability of the former one. What might his unpredictability mean? How many times would I need to explain to him where he was?

And what about managing his physical health? Dad had been diagnosed as diabetic in his 70s. He managed it with oral medications and diet. He showed me his journal where he recorded his sugar levels: "See where it went up here? I had a glass of wine the night before." He had managed his diabetes so well for a long time. But was he a brittle diabetic now, at 89? Would he be able to walk around safely?

Most uncertain of all was the future of his mental state. Could we wrap our heads around the idea that he wouldn't return from where he was?

After a few days in the hospital, Dad's medical condition improved. His diabetes medications were adjusted, his infection gone, and he was eating at regular intervals. At that point, we looked to transfer him to another nursing home for rehabilitation. Laurie had been researching nursing homes. She discovered that the place Dad had been—while it had looked beautiful—had several citations for allowing patients to become dehydrated. The family decided on a different nursing home, with excellent marks, and Dad was admitted there.

I admit to being a little crazy during the time Dad was transferring to the new rehabilitation place. I read the Valentine's Day letter to the nurses and doctor on the floor, so they could hear for themselves that just four weeks before, my father had been an "extraordinarily appropriate," mentally strong man. I missed my father's more familiar way of interacting. But despite the expressiveness and eccentricities of this new man, I could still recognize my father. I continued to find his warmth and love a welcome blanket in my life.

Chapter 3
Engaged and Disconnected

The new nursing home was not beautiful, like the previous one, but it was clean. Pictures of the elected officers among the residents hung immediately inside the front door. Pictures of each resident hung outside the rooms. This nursing home was set up to deliver medical services, with several nurses' stations. Residents were not deposited in front of the televisions as in the other facility. Instead, nurses and nurse's aides paused to interact with the residents, and occasionally even gave them a hug or kiss. They tended to the needs of each person as an individual. Their activities focused on the patients. These people had a sense of mission about their work. Dad responded with gratitude for their gentle kindness.

This nursing home also changed his diagnosis. The working hypothesis was that he had had a stroke. Here, through therapy, he could work to recover his motor skills, relearning how to eat, speak, and walk. His days were busy with therapies: physical, speech, and occupational. Eventually, he would "graduate" to the memory care unit, where he would receive additional special care.

I was scheduled to start teaching an acupuncture class in Hollywood, Florida, so with great reluctance, I left. Jan called me whenever she visited Dad in the nursing home, so we all could talk together. On one of these calls, I received one of many unexpected gifts.

Dad asked this question: what were my acupuncture students searching for when they chose this type of work? I thought it a wonderful question from a man toward the end of his life, looking for meaning. This was the more familiar father, the person I longed for. When I went back into the classroom, I explained that I had just been speaking with my "demented" father, and he had asked a question, which I then posed to them. Through his curiosity, he was able to stimulate other people's insight. The students responded with a wonder and an openness that my father still managed to generate.

I hadn't always been close with my father. I hadn't always appreciated him. Mostly Dad and I argued. From the time I was little, I asserted my independence. We couldn't find the rhythm to meet each other and listen. He was stubborn. I was stubborn. He had all the authority. I felt I had to fight him.

In my 20s, I was committed to making changes in society. I felt strongly that by working with organizations offering health care at free clinics, or counseling at Rape Crisis centers, that we could change society and the ways in which health services functioned in this country.

Dad challenged my opinions. When I decided to go to acupuncture school, he questioned whether this was a reasonable choice. "Can you make a living?" he asked. In his hearts of hearts, I think he wanted me to be happy, but he didn't understand my perspective and couldn't see the destination I was heading toward. He had always kept his nose to the grindstone, supporting his family. I was searching for a different life. We couldn't find each other in these conversations. We didn't know how to listen to each other.

But we had been in this place of illness and crisis before. In 1984, when I was in acupuncture school, Dad had a heart attack and needed double bypass surgery. I received the news that he was waiting in the hospital and would have surgery the next day. I was reluctant to go to be with my family. We always clashed. I didn't want it to be this way. I also didn't want to go there and make a difficult moment in my family worse. I spoke with a friend, who encouraged me to go despite my reluctance. I was going to be there for my entire family, and for myself.

When I arrived at the hospital the next day, I found my mother in the cardiac recovery waiting room, very anxious. She had seen Dad, but he was allowed visitors for only 10 minutes every two hours. I thought that at least I could help her feel better.

When visiting time came, we went in. Dad was alert and trying to accommodate a nurse who needed him to move his arm. He had an array of tubes he was connected to, including one in his mouth.

He saw me and registered a mild look of surprise. Then he wrote on a pad of paper: "What airline did you fly in on?"

I answered: "Piedmont." It was a regional carrier with slightly cheaper fares.

"Good," he wrote.

I thought, *Great. Here he is hooked up to machines and he's focused on whether I spent $35 more getting here. What a f------ asshole. He can't even be present for his own life-threatening situation.*

Then I remember thinking that it was all absurd anyway. I looked at him with the tubes coming out of his mouth, with IVs attached to him, with the constant beeping of the monitors behind him. I walked closer to him and took his hand in mine and held it. A few minutes before, I had been cursing Dad, and now I felt an unstoppable wave of sympathy for him. He caught my attention and looked me straight in the eyes. I saw a softness in his eyes that I had never seen before. And I felt a love from his newly repaired heart that I hadn't felt before and was shocked to receive.

I was amazed. Dad was a man who tried to do the right thing all the time. There was something noble, stable, intelligent, and predictable about him. He was supportive, but I always thought it was very automatic with him. I didn't know his heart, and at that point in 1984, we seldom talked about his feelings.

I felt this connection and realized my father's love for me. I was so overwhelmed that I started to faint.

There were no words. I knew he cherished me despite our past difficult interactions. On this medical unit, they were used to seeing people faint from the stress of seeing loved ones in dire circumstances and connected to machines. And here I was feeling love—and finding myself sitting in a chair with my head between my legs.

My mother, who was already uncomfortable and anxious, began screaming at me: "Evie, *shtarka, mein shtarka!*" (Yiddish for "my strong one.") "What are you doing? Stop that."

I remember thinking: *Wait until I tell her what I felt. She'll understand then. Maybe she'll be happy that Dad and I won't fight so much.*

Dad recovered well, and I returned home to Washington, D.C., within a few days. I called him and talked with him about how significant it was for me to know that he loved me.

He said that he had always loved me and tried to express it as best he could. But we fought so much, and I was stubborn. He did not remember the visits in recovery. But he was glad we could be on better terms.

People who saw our relationship over the next 20 years assumed that my Dad and I had always had an openness and sweetness in our communication. I explained that 30 seconds of feeling love had allowed us to see and listen to each other for the first time. I learned that day that I had a father I could trust. If two bull-headed people like Dad and I could transform how we related and learn to be friends, then anything was possible.

Now, with this latest crisis, it was not only my father who was in transition. We all were. We could not discount Dad in any way, as his confusion at this point seemed limited to a part of his mind that had to do with perceiving and interpreting time and place. He was still interested and curious about the world around him. He wanted to be in charge as he had always been. He was humorous at times and consistently engaged in conversation.

Yet as I observed his work with the speech therapist, I began to understand that he could no longer retrieve basic information. It was startling. For instance, my father had had a gift with numbers. Even when he was 85, I would say to a friend, "Watch this: Dad, what is 27 times 54?" Seconds later, he had the correct answer.

Now, when the speech therapist asked, "Who would you call if the water pipes break and there is a leak?" he didn't have an answer. "Where could you buy a new toothbrush if you lost your toothbrush?" He said if he was without a toothbrush that he could use a piece of wood. I wondered if he would be able to answer if I asked what 3 times 10 is. I did not want to test him.

The therapist also helped Dad learn to eat again, using cards that reminded him to chew and swallow. Just thinking about it was enough to fill me with sorrow. We take these mundane things for granted although they help us manage basic tasks for ourselves and live safely and independently. I wondered how could he have lost so much, so quickly.

Basic aspects of Dad's personality remained intact. Being well organized was very important to him. For most of his life, he made to-do lists before he went to bed. He wanted everything done properly. I admit that I often found this quality useful, but tiresome. In the nursing home, he still needed to get the show organized. He needed to know how things were and how they could be improved. If something were wrong, how would we make it right? He kept all his get-well cards in a brown envelope, which he kept tabs on. Some writing on the envelope made no sense to me, but it was in list format. He was still interested in exerting some control over his environment.

Dad liked to call meetings to get the organization working better. Once I heard an aide saying that Reuben had called a meeting in five minutes. Three or four people gathered in his room. His focus was limited, so he talked for five minutes, laid down the law, recommended changes, encouraged them, and ended the meeting hoping that everything would be straightened out and that things would run much better. It had been 25 years since he had been a merchandise manager of a large department store, working in the role of training and supervision. It was only in watching him in his talks to the staff that I could witness how encouraging and demanding my father must have been as a supervisor. These meetings in his room lasted for a few minutes—and, God love them, the staff at this nursing home were open not just to participating, but also to committing to getting the organization on track.

Unfortunately, in this early stage of this disease, Dad was himself aware of how confused he was. He looked for the nurse and asked her, time and time again, "Shauna, tell me the truth. Am I crazy? I want the truth now." And she would have to tell him that no, he wasn't crazy. During my visits it wasn't unusual for him to look me in the eyes and say: "I'm so confused."

I would say, "It's okay, Dad."

My father's reality continued to shift. The nursing home called us one day to tell us that he had used a water spray in the bathroom to wash all the walls and the beds in his room. The nurse noticed a stream of water running down the hall. They hurried to assume control of the situation. They asked Dad what he had been doing. He just looked away. They asked him again. Finally, he started laughing. He was playing with the water. He was having fun. He was again in the role of a mischievous child pushing the limits that someone else set in a situation, which he no longer understood or controlled. No harm had come in that moment. But I wondered: How could we ever take him home?

Sometimes I arrived early, hoping to see him just after breakfast, and found him fast asleep. I was surprised to find him in bed midmorning. It was so unlike him. When I asked the nurses why he was sleeping during the day, they told me that he wandered the halls all night. He was switching the days for nights. But at this nursing home, they didn't force him to stop the wandering; they gave him time to adjust to his new surroundings. And the aides on night duty talked with Dad as long as he wanted.

Something more was happening for him on a spiritual level. I phoned him every morning and we spoke for 20 minutes. Then I continued my morning meditation, sending him messages about sickness, life, and love. With my mind, I told him that there was nothing to be afraid of, that he was and would always be a part of the universe and a loving part of my heart.

One day during a visit in April, just a month after he had been in this new nursing home, I brought him one of his favorite meals, a chopped chicken liver sandwich from a local deli, and we went in to the family room to enjoy a private lunch. He turned to me and with a somewhat puzzled face, said: "So you die, and then I die, and then we come back?"

I was stunned to hear this. This does reflect some of my beliefs but it did not reflect the exact content of my prayers and messages that I had been sending to him on a daily basis. I had a spiritual practice for decades that combined meditation and prayer. In my family, growing up, when we lit the Sabbath candles every Friday night, we prayed for the health and well-being of people who were struggling. I never lost that impulse to pray. Daily, I would meditate, then pray for people.

I tried to give my father an answer. "First of all, I'm sure that you will die and then I will die. And I believe that yes, we often come back. But we'll see whether or not we see each other again, won't we?"

He turned back to his sandwich and said, "Okay." He was satisfied.

We live in a world that often doesn't allow us to acknowledge the extent of our spiritual connection to each another. I never doubted the spiritual connection I had with Dad, but now I had the gift of knowing how direct all our thoughts and prayers can be. I felt blessed that he could now receive information and loving messages from me that posed a challenging conversation before. Now he would have a new way of being in the present and in the past. There was a lightness and permeability in Dad's ability to receive kindness, love and information. We didn't have to say everything. We communicated all the time.

Dad was on a journey. Understanding his situation was a constant inquiry. And many times I wondered whether a condition was life-threatening or an indication of deterioration. If so, we needed to talk about death. He always claimed that he was not afraid of death. I believed him. He was with us doing loving and kind acts, though in a way far different from any other time in his life. And in some rare moments, I found him to be happy.

Chapter 4
Romeo

The staff at the nursing home nicknamed Dad "Romeo." He often asked one of the nurses if she would marry him. While being given a helping hand around his waist from the occupational therapist, he would allow his hand to slip to her buttocks, where he gave a surprise squeeze. She laughed, and she learned to watch for his hands.

This was not the quiet man that I had known for 49 years. I had to consider that maybe I just didn't know this part of him. I would have described him as your garden-variety, repressed but loving family man, with good Midwestern values. But in this facility, he was receiving intense support and caring relationships all day long. He appreciated every minute of it. And he responded in unanticipated ways.

My niece and brother told me that Dad became immediately infatuated with his 30 something-year-old speech therapist. When I saw him with her, he behaved appropriately, but he told Laurie that he was afraid that she was interested in him. Laurie asked him why he thought this.

Dad answered, "Well, she asked so many personal questions."

"For example?" she asked.

Dad said, "Like whether I was married, and for how long? What has it been like for me to be Jewish?"

In reality, these questions were much more personal than asking, "How are you feeling today, Mr. Soldinger?" And considering that he didn't often know exactly where he was, it might feel at least odd.

He insisted that he was sure the therapist was in love with him.

He asked Laurie's husband, Scott, whether he might know someone closer to his therapist's age, who would be more appropriate for her. Dad was taking steps out of concern for this young woman. His kindness was spilling forward, even if his perception was somewhat misguided.

When the opportunity arose, I repeated the story to the speech therapist. She was already well aware of Dad's infatuation. She laughed and said it was hearts like Dad's that kept her doing the work that she does.

Once when my sister and I were visiting in his room, he looked at me and said, "I don't know how you feel, but the thing that I miss the most is lying next to a person."

He said to me, "It would be okay if you came over and lay down."

I wasn't shocked, and yet I was totally shocked. Dad was always affectionate but never inappropriate. He never intimated anything at all lewd or off-color, and especially not in front of "the girls." He objected if anyone else did, even if we "girls" were in our 40s, and we ourselves might be guilty of making such comments. Yet here he was, asking for me to come over and be affectionate with him in a way that was, to say the least, different.

I tried to receive his comment without judgment and with a soft heart. I went over to him and gently told him, that no, I wouldn't lie down with him, but I embraced him and put my arm around his shoulder.

He was so small. I kissed his forehead. I remembered all the times he had put his arm around my shoulders in a fatherly way, reassuring me when I was afraid or insecure. At that moment I had to get up and ask one of the nurses to help him to the bathroom. When I returned, my sister told me that she also had received that same special invitation, once I left the room.

As Jan and I walked down the hall to leave, we looked at each other, and there was a long pause. What could we say to each other? What words would be comforting? We broke the silence by laughing. The father we had known was gone. His appropriate behavior and conservative ways were out the window. His strong sense of what was proper wasn't as important as feeling loved. So we joked; I looked at my sister and said, "Little girl, want some sugar?" We needed to laugh.

Another day, Dad urgently asked to have a private talk with me. I felt my expectations rising, thinking that we were going to have the talk that all children wait for, about how important different aspects of life are, and how misguided we all are, or how he was looking forward to the time he had left, or how he realized that he was getting better and recovering his faculties. I really wanted him to have an unanticipated change, to wake up from his illness. I wanted to have him back. I took him in the wheelchair to the family visitation room.

"Okay, so what is happening?" I asked.

His shoulders were bent over, and he hardly could look up at me. He said, "Eve, I'm such a bastard."

I protested, "Daddy, why do you say this?" Now, I was filled with fear. What kind of confession might I hear?

He said: "Last night, I fucked a black whore." And then, after a long pause, he continued, "I'm such an SOB."

I didn't know whether to laugh or cry. Sometimes you want to do both. I looked at him crying, held in a wheelchair by a soft restraint, wearing diapers underneath his pants, and as gently as I could, I said to him: "Daddy, have I ever lied to you?"

He looked up at me with his mouth open. With a tear running down one cheek he said, "No."

"Daddy," I said, "it didn't happen."

"Really?" he asked. He had such overwhelming sadness in his expression.

"Really."

He said, "It seemed so real."

I said again, "Really."

"Is that the demented?" he asked.

"Yes," I said. "I think it is." And I fought back my tears.

I noticed that for him, the veils between dreams and reality had become even thinner. He told me about going to a party where the hostess wanted him to stay and to be her boyfriend. He said that he was a married man. And he emphasized that he was seen as desirable, and it surprised him.

After a few months, these romantic and sexual thoughts stopped being shocking to us.

By the time my father went to the nursing home, my parents had been together for 60 years. Growing up, I thought that they were opposites. My mom was creative, eccentric, intuitive, and unpredictable. She was super-sensitive, and discussions or arguments often got viewed as attacks. My father engaged anyone in conversation, had a sense of humor about himself, and was decidedly practical and pragmatic in his approach. He was the parent more curious about other people and their opinions. But both of them were warmhearted, extroverted, and loved the family.

Over the years, I saw a gap widen in their communication. It was easier for each of them to talk to me than it was for them to talk to each other. Each complained to me about the other. I endlessly explained the other person's point of view, and each apologized for saying anything at all to me about what they were feeling. It was stressful to be in that position. But when we were all together we had a familial way of relating, joking and being kind to one another.

Now with this illness, they were even more distant. In the summer of 2004, a year and half since this illness began, my mother ended up in the hospital with congestive heart failure. I took Dad to see her. I had to keep explaining that we were going to visit his wife. He kept correcting me, saying "my former wife." And I repeated, "No, Dad, she is your wedded wife." He found it very confusing.

He said to me, "I'm bewildered about my wife. We don't share a bed."

"No, Dad, because you need special care. You are now living here in this medical unit for people like you with memory problems. But you are still married."

He said to me, "You know I get really confused about who women are, my mother, your mother. They all seem like I can't separate them."

A portrait of the family from the mid-1960s hung on the wall in his room. I showed him each of us and explained the relationships, though I understood that seeing me at 13 years old and in this moment at 50 years old was confusing enough for him. But for the moment, it answered his question and prepared him for his visit with my mother.

When we got to her hospital room, he was charming. He greeted my mother lovingly, asking her how she was feeling. He thanked her for the anniversary card that he had received celebrating their 62nd wedding anniversary, just a few days before. He had rediscovered it on his dresser earlier that day, and thought it was lovely. Within a few minutes after thanking her for the card, he was telling her that he was interested in finding a woman in her 50s to be with. My mother managed not to get upset with him.

We both asked him what he would do with a woman in her 50s.

And his reply was certain: "I'll figure out something."

And then he kissed my mother good-bye, and said that he hoped she would be released from the hospital soon.

◇

Earlier in that year, shortly after he had "graduated" to the memory care unit, we were sitting having a cup of coffee, and he turned to me and said, "You know, I'm really beautiful."

"I know."

"Well, I didn't know."

I asked him, "What did you think of yourself?"

He said, "I thought that I was nice, but now I know that I am beautiful."

I found my heart wondering why we sometimes have to lose our minds to discover our own beauty.

It recalled a haiku I love, by Izumi Shikibu:

> *Watching the moon,*
> *I knew myself completely,*
> *No part left out.*

Now he knew that part too.

Chapter 5
The 90th Birthday Party

As a rule, our family underplayed the importance of birthdays. Large celebrations were few and far between and family reunions infrequent. For my parents' 50th wedding anniversary we had a large party where many of their brothers and sisters came together. Birthdays were celebrated with a family dinner. But now, with Dad's health in question, we realized this was our opportunity to do things differently.

In March and April of 2003, we immersed ourselves in planning a big party for Dad's 90th birthday, in May. Dad was a serious planner. This was his opportunity to have the family and friends get together for a long-anticipated celebration. He wanted to have some input and control over the various parts of the festivities.

During my April visit, Dad got out some paper and a pen to write down the invitation list and to note the time for different activities: hors d'oeuvres at 5:30, dinner at 7, and then dancing. He wanted to discuss the venue for the event, and I told him that Laurie was handling those arrangements. This was the first time in my experience that Dad wasn't in charge. It remained difficult for him to give up control, even if sometimes he wasn't able to complete a thought. All the same, we thought that it would be great to have a big celebration. We worried about it possibly being his last birthday. And we were happy that at least he had something to look forward to.

A few days before the party, I got a call that Dad had fallen. The medical staff were concerned that he had experienced a subdural hematoma—a collection of blood on the surface of the brain after a blow to the head. Dad, who was unable to speak, was taken by ambulance to a hospital. They did a CT scan. By evening, he was transferred to the University of Florida's hospital neurology department, in Gainesville, about two hours from Orlando.

I decided that if the doctors were to perform surgery on my 89-year-old father, I wanted to be there when decisions were being made. Within 20 minutes I had purchased a ticket from California to Orlando for the next morning. On my way to the airport, I received a call from Jan. She said that Dad had asked to talk with me. My first thought was that I wasn't going to make it, and he needed to say goodbye, but then I realized that she said that he had talked. He couldn't speak the day before.

So I placed a call. I first spoke with his nurse who said that he was well, talking, disoriented (as usual), and his symptoms from the night before were rapidly improving. Then Dad got on the phone, and speaking slowly, asked when I would get there. I told him I was on my way to the airport.

With great clarity he said, "Listen. Don't come now. You have to work. Come when you are supposed to come."

I said, "Are you sure? I'm almost to the airport now. I could be there by the end of the day."

He was very clear that it wasn't necessary.

I said, "Good. I'll be there before your 90th birthday."

Three days later, he was transferred back to the nursing home.

Every month had a moment or incident that felt like it might turn into a crisis. When I made plans, I never knew whether I could follow through with them or would soon be racing across the country. I never knew for sure whether I would have the focus or the energy to complete a task. My entire schedule might be on hold only to find out that a problem was not as serious as it seemed at first. Yet every time the alarms went off, I quickly responded—because the alarms always could mean life or death.

Family and friends arrived just before May 6, 2003, my father's 90th birthday. On the day of the party, I brought him some nice clothes to wear for the evening. When I came to pick him up, I found him dressed, in his wheelchair in the hallway, holding onto the rail, and crying.

"Dad, sweetie, what is it?"

The nurse, seeing him distraught, also asked: "Reuben, what is wrong?"

It took him a while to be able to reply through the tears. When he was able to get the words out, he said, "I thought I was dead." He looked traumatized.

"Dad, you aren't dead."

And he said, "Well, I should be dead."

He looked really sad. I was exasperated. So much of my energy, my niece's, brother's, and sister's energy had gone into planning this event. We so wanted to have a celebration of Dad and to give him love and honor and have him feel appreciated. And here he was in the hallway in emotional turmoil. I had to get him out of this. The only way was to treat it as a mood, not get swayed by it, and get him on our schedule if I could.

First, I gave him a big hug and told him, "It is actually a big day. Your wife, kids, grandchild, and great-grandchildren are gathering to celebrate your birthday. It is going to be a great evening. Whenever you will die, it is not going to be this evening, as we already have plans. Now come on. Let's get you ready for your big night ... the celebration of your 90th birthday."

With the help of aides, I got him into the car. I reminded him of everyone who would be there, including my brother, my sister and brother-in-law, Mom, and me. My niece was bringing all of the great-grandchildren, and he would get to see the 2½-year-old twins, Ellie and Emmy, and their little brother, Dylan. And our friends from Jacksonville would be there, and friends from his work from long ago.

It had been only two months since the ER doctor told us Dad didn't have two months to live. We wanted this to be an evening of celebration, not a long goodbye. Yet everyone found it hard to escape the thought that this might be his last birthday.

We celebrated in a beautiful private banquet room in an Italian restaurant. It was a comfortable setting for all, even the little children, who wandered around the room. Dad recognized everyone in attendance. And while he no longer had the same authority, he was basking in the love he felt all around him.

The gifts showed the givers had chosen them with great thought and care. He received two stars registered in his name, two robes, and a picture of him standing with his friends from work. The most important gift was a "memory book" that my niece put together, of photos and stories of his marriage, children, grandchildren, and great-grandchildren. Even a year later, he believed it was the best book and remained amazed at Laurie's ability to have put it together. The book really helped him to stay connected to his relationships with his family and with his past.

My brother made a speech and each of us said a few words around the table of 20 or so family and friends. Dad even spoke for a while about getting together on such occasions in the future. He seemed a few shades paler than usual but continued to enjoy the party.

One of the more poignant moments came as people said their farewells. The wife of one of his work buddies came over and said goodbye. And Dad stood up from his wheelchair with almost Herculean effort. I asked him why he was getting up. He said that he had to see Mrs. McLaughlin to her car. I reassured him that she was fine and that she was with Mr. McLaughlin.

At the birthday party Dad was toasted, watched his great-grandchildren taking piggyback rides, ate a filling and rich meal, and blew out the lights on his birthday cake one more time. And it all went off without a hitch. Well, mostly—as one lovely woman in her late 40s came to say goodbye, the presence of her attractive body got a spontaneous, "We have to see if those are real" from Dad.

Jan and I drove Dad back to the nursing home and I called ahead to let them know to expect us at the entrance. His favorite aide came to help get him from the car. She helped lift him up to get him back in the wheelchair and talked with him about the party. To avoid having to lift him as "dead weight," she asked him to dance with her. It felt appropriate, that he should have some dancing on this special evening. He danced his way into the wheelchair. I went with him to his room and placed the robes and pictures there. He showed the aides the memory book, which include a photo of him in his Army uniform. "You were a handsome man in your uniform," they told him. We gave the staff the leftover cake and left, knowing that he was in excellent, loving hands.

Chapter 6
Having a Future

When I returned to California after the birthday celebration, I was exhausted, and I had caught a little head cold. As I lay in bed, drifting between being awake and asleep, a surprising observation surfaced: I identified with Dad.

I, too, was confused. I was not sure where I was or where I was going. I felt ungrounded in California. A year and a half before I had moved there for a relationship that went sour, and now I was in the midst of a mid-life crisis centered on what I wanted to do for the rest of my life.

What am I doing here? I asked myself. *What is my life purpose?* The fast and easy answer was that I am a healer. But what was the missing link that prevented me from taking action, from going forward? I didn't have those answers. I only had the questions. It was my heart's desire to help others and make a difference. Now, I wondered, what would be the form of the help I provided to others?

And these weren't the only questions I asked myself about how I wanted to live my life. I wanted a devotional spiritual life. I wanted to know myself better. I wanted to create a loving relationship. Feeling lost and uncertain, never before had I had so many questions. I had had my very full acupuncture practice for decades. It was always challenging but felt natural and fulfilling. I felt spiritually guided. I learned to love my clients. I nurtured and felt nurtured by the healing environment. People came for sessions to find their center, to heal all kinds of pain, and to realize their spiritual life. I had a spiritual community. I had a social life. After planting trees in the garden, I enjoyed finding new growth each spring. I loved nature, people, and God. And I was grateful for every moment.

Yet at the age of 49, in this very different moment of my life, I was not sure of anything. I wasn't sure where I wanted to live. And I wasn't sure that I could plant my roots in California. Where was my path? What would my future be? What should I do next? I floundered, having not asked myself these questions for a long time. I was uncertain, not wanting to go backwards. My life involved looking for guidance, praying, grieving my dad's losses, celebrating his presence, grieving a relationship, and feeling generally confused about my goals.

Dad's goals were uncertain, too, and he needed a sense of purpose, just as I did. How could he find it, when every day brought the need to rediscover his basic surroundings? Confusion prevented him from understanding his purpose.

Unlike my dear Dad, I knew how to handle daily life. I was not a danger to myself. I might have been unable to discern a sense of my next steps, but I was certain from a deep place within that much lay ahead in my life, and I had changed directions because it was time.

When I left Orlando after the birthday party, Dad's focus had been on the future. He said that things would get better, and that he wanted me to walk forward in the world with confidence.

Sometimes Dad appeared to be quite normal. I remained hopeful. After all, it had only been two-and-a-half months since his stroke; who knew what might happen? I hoped that the doctors were wrong. He was doing better than many people in similar situations— I could tell that just from looking around the nursing home. I was still not convinced that Dad's dementia was going to get worse.

As I continued to contemplate this, I decided one thing was clear: I was tired of staying in bed nursing this cold.

I needed to get my glasses fixed, so I drove to the optical shop. I called Dad on my way and was surprised to find him agitated. He remembered first to ask me about my cold. Then he said that he was glad that I had called, and he wanted to talk with me.

"Eve, listen to me," he said. "If the doctor can't get me better, then I want to die in the next few minutes, and I want you to help me. I don't want to die in days or in months. I want to die right now."

It was upsetting to hear him so disturbed, demanding, and wanting to end it all. I had to remember the kind of person he is at his core and not become too soothing, but instead to be direct and honest. I remembered resisting my own feelings of heartbreak and speaking with my logical mind:

"Listen, Dad, when it is your time, you will die. Some people get to live four years and some live 84 years. That's just the way it is. And here you are, 90 years old, and continuing to live life. You get to enjoy your great-grandchildren and the beautiful days. I promise you that you will die, and when you die, you will do it just perfectly and beautifully, at the right time."

As if I had said magic words, he became calmer. "I'm happy with that answer," he said. "You're a great woman."

I said, quietly, "You are a great man."

I didn't know how I persuaded him away from his objective, but I knew that he understood enjoying and engaging in life. Yet I needed to do something more. I called Craig and told him about the conversation. He said that he would make sure to visit Dad the next day.

Was this a post-birthday depression, or just a naturally occurring depression that came from his awareness of being somewhat better, though never the same? We worried Dad would lose his sense of the future, while he was still so engaged with us. And we were worried about what promise the future had for him. I knew that even if I stayed in my own confusion for a while, with a seemingly uncertain future, that I still held a belief that life would calm down, things would change, and I would find my way. I had faith in this. And while Dad often didn't know where he was, he maintained his place as an encouraging, supportive, and present parent. Now he needed our encouragement.

But it was difficult to switch roles. Dad started conversations, as always, by asking "What's new?" Sometimes I exaggerated the reports of my progress. He kidded with me, saying something like, "I knew you could do it, even if you didn't."

Though his faith in me was seemingly endless, I couldn't let him know how much of my time I spent processing my reactions to his illness and deterioration. It was not in keeping with what he would have hoped.

So I asked him how he was. He told me that he was getting out of there on Sunday and going home. He felt that he had been "negligent" of his responsibilities.

I explained to him that that was not a remote possibility. I said, "You have taken care of everything for us, and we appreciate it, and now you can relax. The future is good. You have made great progress. You have to keep working in therapy."

"Yes, I am getting much stronger from doing all the therapies. Maybe your mother should be getting these kinds of sessions."

"What you really need is for this once, at least in the short term, to focus on yourself, and get stronger. This is your job."

Although he agreed, it was like swimming against the current. Not even dementia could allow him to be a different person. He wanted to always assure the future for his loved ones and to create every kind of stability in our lives. In his world, he was in charge of safeguarding our future. Keeping to the plans had become his way of focusing on the future. And now his future always held new uncertainties.

For the present, I chose to celebrate life with him even with confusion. And I chose to accept confusion as a sometimes companion in life, no matter what my age.

Chapter 7
Fears and Illusions

Dad had always liked keeping to a schedule. As the weeks flowed into months, I developed a routine for our contact, too. Jan and I visited Florida on alternating months, and sometimes I stayed a week or longer. I spoke to the nurses once a week about how he was doing, and checked in with Jan and Craig often.

Prior to his illness, Dad and I might have had a long phone conversation once a month, and shorter conversations once a week. My sense of connection with him was a given.

But now that he was disoriented, I did my best to call everyday. I got up, meditated, and, while walking my dog, called him on my cell phone. It would be 7:15 a.m. in California and a convenient time to reach him on the East Coast. The nurses told me that he waited at the nurse's station at that hour, predicting each call would be his daughter.

Yet once we began talking, nothing was routine. There was no way of knowing where he would think he was, or what his story might be.

Often the first words out of his mouth were: "How did you find me?"

And I replied, increasingly with nonchalance, "Where are you?"

"Eve, I'm at the police station. I am accused of selling drugs. I'm going to jail. I'm so sorry. I brought all this shame on the family."

What should I say? Should I burst his reality wide open? Should I ask him what kind of drugs, when I'm sure he had never touched, seen, or experienced an illicit drug in his life? Why this? Did this question represent something in him psychologically? Did this go to some untapped fear? Dad had never even gotten a speeding ticket. Was this the unmarked territory of the dementia? Would he find a means to experience any shame in his consciousness that needed healing?

I chose to be reassuring. "Dad, I know all about it, and we just need to straighten a few things out, and everything is going to be okay. You are not going to jail. I promise that we are going to get this straightened out."

Sometimes he reported being held prisoner in a police station. Once he was there "for stealing $1,000." Should I tell him that his reality was an illusion? I told him that he had been falsely accused, and there was no theft. No charges were pressed, and he was free to go.

Once he regretted having to tell me that his twin great-granddaughters had been kidnapped, but were now okay. He assured me that it had been very scary. It felt like he experienced fears that he might never have imagined. His survival and the survival of all his loved ones were major concerns. His life did not have a sense of safety or security.

"Oh, Eve, how did you find me?"

"Dad, I can always find you. Where are you right now?"

"I'm in New York at a hotel and waiting to have brunch with my brothers."

"Is it a nice hotel?" I asked.

"Very nice."

"Which brothers are you meeting?"

He said: "Nate and Oscar. They are putting on a big spread. You know, Nate owns all this real estate here. He has made a fortune."

I didn't want to tell him that Nate and Oscar had already passed over. I thought maybe they were making more contact with him. And I liked the idea that in some dimension of time, my uncles were present to Dad.

"Are many other people coming?"

"Yes, there's a large crowd." He added, typical of him: "Listen, we'll call you as more of us come together. Thanks for calling."

Or there was a more disturbing reality:

"Eve, I'm so glad you found me. I'm in a park where Craig left me, and I don't have any money to get back home."

"Daddy, stay right where you are and I'll make sure that Craig comes to pick you up. Okay?"

And he repeated, "Okay."

He was inside a health care facility feeling lost and alone. I couldn't just say that wasn't true. It wasn't that way. So I lied. I said that he would be rescued. I said that the family would save him. I also knew that within an hour after a meal or a nap that he was likely to realize he was in a very different place. He would engage in conversations with some other people there. And the question of whether or not he would be saved would be long gone. There would be a whole new set of circumstances for him to discern.

"Eve, oh, I'm so glad you called. I have bad news."

"What?"

"It's Craig. He had a terrible accident, and I can't find him. It's been days since anyone heard from him."

"No, Dad. I spoke with Craig and he is just fine."

"When did you speak with him?" he asked.

"Last night."

"I am so relieved. I've been so upset."

Once during a visit, he told me that he had gone out with some of the other residents the night before and that he had needed to borrow $50 to take a cab to get home. And he had promised to return the borrowed money by noon, and he didn't have a dollar in his pocket.

I was very interested in what kind of night on the town he had. "So where were you?"

"Oh, we went to a club. There were all kinds of people there. Whites, African Americans, Asians, gays, Jews, all kinds."

"Did you have a good time?" I asked.

"Yes, but I said that I would return the money by noon to Ray. You know him, don't you?"

"Yes, I know him. (I actually believed that Ray was Rae, one of the female health care workers. Dad had taken her name for this remembrance.) Dad, I'll take care of it. I promise. You can trust me.

Fifty dollars by noon. I'll take care of it right after our visit."

He said, "Thank you so much. I was worried. I have no money. What kind of man doesn't have a dollar in his pocket?"

Later as I was leaving, he looked at me and wagged his finger in the air, saying, "Remember, you promised."

Here he was, not able to distinguish reality from fantasy, and yet not willing to shirk his responsibilities.

For my mother, the occasions when he shared such fears were some of the most difficult conversations. My father had always been a rock of firmness and stability. She had always been the person with creative grandiose ideas, writing poems, performing in plays, and directing musicals. When we were young, she was immersed in being an attentive mother in very creative ways. When she wasn't engaged creatively, she might sink into a depression of a few days or weeks.

As an adult, I eventually realized that she suffered from undiagnosed bipolar disorder. When we were in high school, if she sank into a depression, Jan and I took care of her. She might be in bed for days. My father didn't realize her difficulties until we left for college and were no longer available to be caregivers. Once he understood the situation, he wrote me a letter apologizing for the burden we had shouldered at home.

My mother was sensitive and wise. She understood many things about her children and offered great advice to me, but coping with her husband's illness was too challenging for her. She retreated when his world didn't match ours. If she visited, she left the facility crying and continued crying for an entire day and night. Her visits became less frequent as his condition deteriorated. She visited him reluctantly every few months.

My brother's approach was to always tell him the truth and felt that in a way he became the bad guy. He would tell Dad, "No, that's not what happened." He did it well. Dad often was calmed by his reality checks. -

Craig wrote Dad this letter so that he would have the facts close at hand.

Hi Dad,

I'm writing this letter to help you understand reality a little better. February 21, 2002, you had a mini stroke that left you with dementia (which is a condition leaving you with a bad memory and lots of confusion). Since then we've only been able to care for you by having you in a nursing facility. This is the third place you've been … and the best. It's called Ivy Court and you've been here nearly a year.

Your daughters, Eve and Jan, visit often to help make sure you're doing well. You're in Orlando … and are near where Laurie and Scott and the babies live … and also close to where I live … and where I take care of your wife, Florence (Mom).

You haven't been to New York in nearly 30 years ... and haven't left and been outside on your own in two years.

You're not leaving there and moving anywhere for some time ...

Dad, everyone loves you and is doing all we can to get you the best care possible. We want you to be able to enjoy your family as best you can and as often as you can.

He wrote the letter to be helpful, but Dad didn't think to read it when he was confused. And when he did read it, very little time passed before he forgot again.

My sister tended, as I did, to think that there was some deeper meaning to every scene in which my father found himself. Often, we risked going there with him.

I wondered how frightening the world was becoming to him. I wondered how powerfully wedded we become to our reality, and whether there wasn't something important to be gained from the reality that Dad was experiencing. His world was subject to alternate interpretations, but his was not a separate world.

In some fleeting moments of clarity, Dad realized that he had lost his grasp on reality. I wondered what he would have said about himself, if he were the observer. "Poor fellow, he's lost his marbles. He was such a fine man. It's a shame." Or would it be more personal: "Oh my God, what has happened to me? What kind of garbage am I saying?"

I only knew that having a different sense of reality didn't lessen our ability to see the reality of each other. I recognized his fears and reassured him. He was always thankful to know that his deepest fears were not true, and that his imagined situations were not as dire as they appeared to be. Every one of us desires a friend who can calm our deepest fears. He was no different. His world was not a separate world, but it was not a stable world. His world changed for him at any given moment. Never before had he needed our reassurance. Instead, he had always been the one to reassure us. But now we found him in fear, and we responded with the kindness that we had always known from him. Now we changed roles and reassured him that all was well and that we would take care of things that he could no longer do. We now knew his fears.

Chapter 8
My Moral Compass

My father was a just man. He summed up people by their character and by what they were willing to stand up for. He was passionate about doing the right thing, whether that meant finishing a project or making political decisions. When he had an opinion, he had to take action. From him, I learned how it was possible to determine my own moral ground.

I was a 5-year-old when we moved from the Midwest to Jacksonville, Florida. Dad became the manager of a large downtown department store. He saw that there were "whites only" signs on the bathrooms and quickly made an executive decision to take them down. This was in 1959, a short time before civil rights protests became more visible. Dad took this action with no fanfare. There were no reports in the news. He did it when the store was closed at the end of the day. He had no idea what it would mean to take this action.

From the stories that my mother told, it meant quite a lot. We received numerous phone calls, and whoever answered the phone was called racist, hateful names. Because I was a child at the time, I don't remember the calls, but I learned who my father was and that individual action was always important. I learned the power of taking action even if the results are unpopular. It had a huge influence on how I make decisions in my life and how I take stands.

Dad was an army captain in World War II; he won the Silver Star and two Bronze Stars, and French medals as well. Our house had a whole wall covered with framed medals. I never heard the stories that went with the medals. Dad hated braggarts. He was a part of a generation of humble men. A year into his illness, he mentioned how he never talked about his medals, and he didn't know why, though he could recall that he didn't like boasting.

In the late 1960s, Charles de Gaulle made statements Dad considered anti-American—coupled with policies Dad considered anti-Semitic. So my father sent his framed French medals to the French Embassy, saying that these awards no longer had value. He often joked that he had never heard back from the French government. We laughed along, but we all understood that the medals had meant something to him.

We were watching the evening news together on the day in 1968 when Columbia University students took over the administration building in protest of the Vietnam War. Dad became infuriated. He burst forward with an angry declaration that if my sister and I ever did such a thing to protest United States policy, he would disown us. The violence of the students combined with the protest against American policy was the antithesis of what he believed to be correct action.

I was in eighth grade at the time and sometimes got into trouble at school for talking too much, but I had never seen anything like this. I was just beginning to absorb the information about the Vietnam War. It bore no resemblance to the suffering during World War II. My father's outburst left me wide-eyed. I was a little frightened, but I didn't worry about what he was declaring. I just saw it as being another moral code that I now had to be aware of: *No taking over college administration buildings to protest U.S. policy.* Got it.

A few years later, in 1971, while I was in high school, Dad read the *Pentagon Papers,* the collection of top secret documents on Vietnam released by Daniel Ellsberg. I remember seeing the book on his nightstand. One night I was in the kitchen helping to prepare dinner, and Dad came in, saying: "Eve, I owe you an apology. I just finished reading the *Pentagon Papers,* and I want you to know that I was wrong about the students at Columbia; they were right to take over the administration building protesting this war. We have absolutely no business being there. I can't believe what a mess we are making. I'm sorry for my outburst before and what I said to you."

There were several things that astonished me about that. For one, he acted as if he had been thinking about his admonition all this time. It had been an event of years past for me. I understood it was a sensitive area of potential heated debate and consciously avoided it. Second, I was astonished that he took this opportunity to correct his opinion and to actually apologize to me. He was willing to say he was wrong. In effect, he was encouraging me to stand up for what I would find to be right and just.

But most important to me was that his statement had to do with the violence we make in the world. I was 17 years old and just beginning to take in the world outside my small, self-conscious, high school view. I was coming to understand how important it was to take action to protest unjust situations. Dad showed me how much he believed in individual action.

Even in the nursing home, he maintained this sense of justice— sometimes with interesting results. He had a habit of wandering the halls in his wheelchair. He stopped to have conversations, mostly with the staff. The group activities offered by the nursing home were not of great interest to him. Instead, he loved engaging in one-on-one conversations. Mostly he was encouraging, appreciative, grateful, and flirtatious. Often, he stayed up much of the night, talking with one or another staff members, until he tired. Much of the time, he would have to concentrate in order to remember where his room was. He would wander into other people's rooms, looking for one of the family or, as he said, stock for the department store. I was with him one day when he wandered into a woman's room. A staff person came to redirect him.

"Now Reuben," she said, starting to turn the wheelchair around, "you know that you aren't allowed in the women's rooms."

He looked up at her surprised, gathered himself to understand the situation for a moment, and hit his fist against the arm of the wheelchair, declaring each word clearly and indignantly: "This prejudice has got to stop. I should be allowed to go anywhere. I will not tolerate it."

I knew this man very well. This part of him remained intact.

I had to turn away. I walked out in the hall, leaned against the wall and began to laugh as quietly as I could manage. I was laughing at the absurdity of Dad finding his righteous indignation at this moment. And in part I was laughing that this was him, my father, making his opinion based on some sense of justice and ultimately, kindness. Even if he had misjudged the situation, I recognized him.

Another time, the nurse called me to say that Dad was agitated. They were having trouble calming him down and couldn't reach my brother. My brother was good at reassuring Dad and calming him down. But I was glad that they had called me.

The nursing home put Dad on the phone. He was ranting: "Eve, Eve. Vice President Dick Cheney has been lying to the American people, and we need to stop this abomination." He started shouting. "It's important, before the Veep destroys the whole country. He is going to take the entire country down. He is lying. We need to organize groups throughout the country to stop this. And we need to do it now!" This was not a discussion. Every word was in the imperative.

The war in Iraq had recently begun. I was opposed to this war, but I didn't know how to help Dad at this moment, except to say that I was working on it and encouraging him to breathe. This was not the best strategy. His moral indignation was profound. He was in the midst of this truth of what we were doing in Iraq. He needed to protect and defend his truth. I wondered: if a so-called "normal" person was so agitated around this issue, would we think that their reaction was out of proportion?

Dad no longer had emotional defenses to cover his intense reactions. And at this moment, he was aware of what was happening with American troops in Iraq. I wondered how the rest of us distill our emotional reactions to the atrocities all over the world until we have no outrage, no moral indignation; until we feel a separateness, from which my father no longer suffered. Though overwhelmed from the intensity of his response, I didn't really think that he was off base. He simply had none of the usual outlets for his feelings and thoughts.

While trying to calm him down, I realized that this moral man was part of my father's essence, his core being, and I didn't want to diminish him or try to invalidate him in any way. So I listened. And I wondered how he had figured out what was happening politically. He could no longer read a paragraph. He didn't understand what was happening when he watched the news. Every once in a while I reminded him to breathe.

All I could do was hope that he would tire and not remain agitated, but I understood that he was speaking with an emotional intensity that was hard to channel. And I didn't think that he was out of his mind. Once again, I was proud of him. Once again, I found myself admiring his integrity. He was still a responsible citizen. In my heart, I promised him that I would stand for all the values that I believe in and purposely move forward toward a compassionate and ethical life, following his passionate and just example.

Chapter 9
Violence

Of all the changes in Dad's behavior, I believe the one that shocked me and my family most was violence. I came to understand this often happens in dementia cases. But the first time Dad experienced such an episode, we were heartbroken.

Dad had been in the nursing home for only four months when Craig called me early one morning with shocking news. Dad had punched a woman in the face, and she had been sent for X-rays. Apparently the incident resulted from a disagreement over wheelchair navigation. My brother tried to joke that if they kicked Dad out of the home, we could put him in the boxing ring.

I was stunned as I put down the phone. My father was a natural peacemaker. He came from a family of six children, and often there were conflicts. Growing up, he lived in a small home, where his parents had one bedroom and the children had the other. When they were small, there were only two beds, one for the boys and the other for the girls. They learned to get along. His mother was a wise woman who handled the conflicts with firmness and compassion.

Dad was much like her. He talked things out and brought harmony among family members. He could see both sides of any situation, and he was sensitive to people's fragility.

My gentle, intelligent, just father, so sensitive to the subtleties of human interactions, now was using violent behavior. Only a few months after his diagnosis, he was faltering in his ability to control any impulses.

Although Dad had had his share of extreme frustrations and great passions, he had no violence in him. He had never hit anyone. As a teenager, I had challenged his authority in most every way. We had many arguments, and my objective was to get him to concede or to get him to laugh about it.

I remember him coming into my room once when I was a senior in high school at a moment when I was angry about some now-forgotten issue. I used a long string of f-words. Dad was angry that I'd used such language and demanded that I stop.

As he reprimanded me, I remember my anger escalating. I turned to him and said defiantly: "Oh, Dad—I'm not *doing* it, I'm just *saying* it." He started to laugh—and had to make a quick exit.

◇

Dad was one to keep his distance from volatile situations. He told me a story about leaving one job where the storeowners were two brothers who used fisticuffs. He refused to be a part of it. The idea of people hitting each other defined the limits of what he would tolerate.

But now my Dad had hit someone. He had hit a woman. She needed X-rays. I called a few of my friends crying, seeking some sense of support in a now-shaky world. I spent much of the day on the phone with the staff of the nursing home or speaking with members of my shocked family.

In the conversation with my brother, he questioned whether this meant that they wouldn't be able to keep Dad at the nursing home. I couldn't focus on the consequences. It was enough to have to absorb the idea that this happened at all. To think that he could actually have hurt another human being was a startling reality. In the end, the woman was fine and didn't sustain any injury. But we now had to worry about what would happen tomorrow or the next day. And of course we thought that if he were home with us, this new impulsive violence could be directed toward Craig, or Mom, or whoever was around.

Just two days before the hitting incident, we had spoken on the phone. Dad said, "Always remember how deeply I love you." He repeated it three times, needing to make sure that he communicated this feeling to me. And he had. I felt that he had lost part of his mind, but had found this enormous heart. With this new violent behavior, I was caught even more off guard.

When the nurse asked him why he had hit the fellow patient, it was as if she were asking about something he knew nothing about. He stared at her with surprise. I tried to imagine what it must have been like for him. Maybe he was so mad he felt like socking her in the face—and then hadn't realized that his thought went from his mind to reality.

How could he not know that he had hit this woman? Was frustration leading him? How could I give him credit for so much he was going through, yet discount the importance of this?

As Craig and I spoke to more staff at the nursing home, it appeared that there had been some provocation. That made no difference. He still socked someone in the jaw. If he no longer had impulse control, what would his life be like? After all, Dad wasn't angry all the time.

A few weeks later, it happened again. He slapped the hand of a resident who tried to move him out of another man's room. Dad had thought he belonged there. If he had realized he didn't belong there, my father, as I had known him, would have politely exited.

Residents were instructed to get a staff person if Reuben wandered into their room. One sweet woman told me that he often wandered into her room looking for his daughter. I'm fairly sure at those moments that he thought he was in a hotel.

I asked a nurse I often spoke to if Dad might be kicked out of the nursing home for being unmanageable. She allayed my concerns, reassuring me that Dad had a caring place. I could continue to trust the staff, from the people who served the meals, to the staff who checked that he was eating, to the nurses and aides who helped him to the bathroom as well as helping him to bed at night. There was one aide who actually sang him a lullaby when she put him down for the evening. He thought that the workers were his friends, though the residents, for some unknown reason, were not.

A few months later, in August, I drove from California to Florida and then to Washington, D.C., to teach a class. On the weekend I taught, I decided not to call Dad. I needed to focus. I told him I wouldn't be calling. Afterwards, when I took to the road for the long trip home to California, I called Craig. He had more shocking news: one of the residents had called the police on Dad for making threats.

I couldn't be hearing right. Maybe it was poor reception with the cell phone. Maybe Craig was speaking an unknown language or code that I couldn't quite interpret. For the first time on my long drive, I pulled over and stopped on the side of the road.

According to the reports of staff and of my father, one of the other residents was using some swear words. Dad got upset; in one retelling, he said that his great-grandchildren were in the room. He told the man that if he didn't stop swearing, he "would knock his block off."

The other resident went to a phone and called 911, reporting that he was being threatened. Two policemen arrived in short order, much to the surprise of the staff. I imagine that the police expected to hear of staff abuse. But they were required to check it out—and ended up speaking with my father—90 years old, confused, in a wheelchair, but unrelenting in his beliefs. I think Dad was very proud that he had been taken seriously. He claimed that he could have knocked his block off, too. And he maintained that the man shouldn't have used that language around women.

I imagined my law-abiding, gentle, Dad, having a first-ever police report made about him. I imagined that the policemen finding themselves in the middle of several elderly patients with dementia, with proposed threats from men in wheelchairs, were probably not going to write up a standard police report.

Mostly what I sensed was a goodbye to yet another familiar and comfortable façade and an acceptance of this new aspect of his personality. Was it his medications? Would Dad misconstrue much of the world in front of him? Would these episodes of violence become more common? We would love him in the midst of it all. I would miss him now, and I hoped that under some circumstances, he might still be a peacemaker.

Chapter 10
Forgiveness

When I was growing up in the 1950s and '60s, every Friday night our family observed the Sabbath with traditional blessings, festive foods, and a spirit of prayerfulness. After the meal, we might go to synagogue; more often we stayed home together and sang Hebrew and Yiddish songs. I cherished the warm, loving atmosphere we created each week. There was a present spiritual life for us as a family.

Also, as post-World War II Jews, we were aware of the catastrophic effects of prejudice in this world. The atrocities of the Holocaust, whether spoken of or not, were present in their effects of generating resentment, anger, and fear within our family.

As a captain with the U.S. Army 8th Infantry Division, Dad was part of the company that liberated the Nazi labor camp Woebbelin, on May 2, 1945. He had original photos from that day. As a teenager, I remembered looking at his photo album and wondering how people could face such things and retain any trust in love, civilization, or goodwill. Dad always identified himself as a Jewish serviceman, and he felt the grief and pain for people who might have been his family. He eventually gave the photos and the negatives to the United States Holocaust Museum, in Washington, D.C.

Fifty years after the end of World War II, he finally began telling us stories of Jewish people he met who had successfully hidden during the war. The 8th Infantry landed in Normandy on July 4, 1944. They fought through to Rennes by July 28th. My father and another officer, Ben Cohen, went to the Prefect of Police to ask whether there were any Jews still living there. The police chief directed them to a family where a child had been hidden. It wasn't until my father and his fellow officer came in and made their inquiry, that the family realized the police had known they were hiding the child and had kept their secret. There, in front of my father, this kind French man who had risked his life hiding a young Jewish girl removed the cross from around her neck, telling her she didn't have to wear it anymore.

Dad was deeply sensitive to discrimination, whether it was against Jews, African-Americans, Latinos, or gay people. However, discrimination against women wasn't as obvious to him, and on several occasions in the late '70s, I provided some education to him on these issues. We had some disagreements, but we learned to listen to one another.

However, he had a blind spot when it came to Germans: He equated them all with the Nazis. He hated seeing people buy anything

German and was infuriated at the popularity of Volkswagen cars in the '60s. The Germans were the enemy in the war, but worse, he said, they slaughtered *our* people. We hardly spoke of Hitler, concentration camps or Nazis, but there was an underlying fear of anti-Semitism, Germans, and governments capable of murder. My mother's version of this was to object if she heard me listening to music by Wagner.

As the years went by, the outbursts about Germans were less frequent, but they were still his strongest-held prejudice.

A few months after Dad entered the nursing home, I was visiting for lunch and saw that there was an after-lunch activity of building World War II models. Some younger residents were making a model of a German Panzer tank. I thought that as a World War II vet, Dad might be interested in this. I put the blueprint of the model in Dad's hands and asked if it was like the real thing. I thought it might bring up memories.

He looked at it pretty carefully and said, "Yes, it actually is identical to the real thing."

I asked him, "Did you ever see one up close?"

And he replied, "Oh, sure. I saw them many times."

I was unsure what the follow-up question would do. I didn't want to make him feel bad. But I went forward anyway.

"Do you remember the last time you saw anything like this?"

"I don't remember."

I spent a few minutes chatting with the other people in the room about how things were going. Dad kept looking at the blueprint and acting as if he was reading about the tank. I thought that he didn't have the capability to read anymore, but I wouldn't stop him from trying. After about 20 minutes, I noticed that while the blueprint remained in Dad's hand his head was nodding forward.

I turned to him and asked whether he wanted to leave, and he said yes. So I got behind the wheelchair, unlocked the brakes, and prepared to move him around the table.

He seemed to want to say something to me, so I bent over so he could speak in my ear. In a very calm and gentle voice, he said: "You know, we were just soldiers on opposite sides of a war. We really weren't different from one another."

I was surprised. This was an unexpected comment. I didn't know whether to take it seriously or whether a moment of heartfelt forgiveness had occurred. I needed a minute to think what to say next.

Before we left the room he turned to the three other people in the room and said, "*Auf Wiedersehen.* We have had a nice visit. Thank you very much. *Bitte schoen.*"

I started to giggle nervously, realizing that he thought we were in Germany.

As I wheeled him back to his room, he stopped one of the aides he knew and shook her hand, saying: "Hello, I'm Reuben Soldinger from Toledo, Ohio. We have been having a great trip. How are you doing?"

While she didn't realize that Dad thought that we were traveling through Germany, she said she was doing just fine, and it was good to see him.

Dad held onto her hand and expressed his hope that she was having as good a time as we were having during this trip.

She didn't understand the context of his comments, but in a seasoned and practiced way focused for a moment, saying: "It's wonderful to have your daughter visiting."

"Oh, yes. We are enjoying our travels." And then he said, *"Auf Wiedersehen."*

He was greeting everyone he saw in German, as if it was the first time he had met them. Then he looked at the walls and said: "Isn't this a beautiful place? What a wonderful hotel."

I gave him a kiss on the cheek. Whether the hotel was beautiful, well … I couldn't see his hotel. I felt pain from realizing he didn't know where he was from one hour to the next. Yet I couldn't help but notice that there was still the possibility of healing his heart and seeing the situation differently and without pain and animosity. He was in Germany and having a good time, offering his hand and heart in friendship. While some people only talk of forgiveness, my father had taken it upon himself to heal this hatred by being in forgiveness with Germans. There was power and consciousness in his process. In this moment Dad visited not just Germany but also a forgiveness that he had never known.

Chapter 11
Kindness and Gratitude

Dad was a listener. His brand of generosity let him take in people during his first interactions with them. If he noticed something in a person's self-esteem was wounded, he tried to say something supportive and fatherly. He always acknowledged a job well done.

During my last visit before his stroke in January, 2003, Dad and I had a poignant conversation about the meaning of life. I had retired one evening and was in the guest bedroom reading a rather esoteric book on acupuncture theory. I welcomed the interruption when Dad knocked on the door. He asked me about the book and I explained the ideas as best I could. "It's really all about understanding what it all means, how things change and why they don't," I said. "It is just about life. Dad, what do you think is important when you assess a life? What is important to do in life?"

Dad was absolutely clear: "The most important thing is what you actually do for people. Eve, as I look back on my life, it's the kindness and effort I have made to help others that I think really counts."

He recalled his mother's funeral, in 1943; there were people in attendance whom he had never met, there because my grandmother had always had a kind word for them. I felt the love that he had always expressed for his mother; it was her open heart that gave meaning to our conversation.

Then Dad spoke of the different people whose lives he felt that *he* had touched and how important being generous was to him. Listening to him, I understood that he was sharing some deep feelings he had about how to live life. But I also thought he had set narrow criteria for judging himself. I wondered. I listened. I thought he was being hard on himself. He was a loving father, a steadfast loyal husband, a true family man, and interested in and curious about the many ways that the world works.

We ended up talking for hours, touching on everything from how to balance the many aspects in life of home and family, to world crises. We indulged in an over-the-top love fest as we shared stories about his three young great-grandchildren, Emmy, Ellie, and Dylan.

At the time, I didn't know that this would be our last serious conversation, the last time we were grounded in the same reality, where the past was still past, and the present a shared experience of events and circumstances.

◇

We had a lifetime of such connections and conversations. No matter what transition I was facing in my life, each month Dad wrote me a letter with some encouraging or hopeful responses. Often, I found notes saved in a favorite book or among my papers, giving me the chance to reread his encouragement. If I traveled to study with a master healer or spiritual leader, he wrote that he hoped that I would find the inspiration that I was seeking. He actually wrote thank you notes after visiting me, saying what a good time he had, and that I should leave more work for him to do around the house so he could help me out. Or he acknowledged that through an acupuncture treatment, or through listening and interacting with him, or Mom, or my brother or sister, that I had contributed my knowledge and understanding to our family. I came to understand through his expressiveness that kindness, generosity, and gratitude are never boring, and that expressing them exercises the brightest part of the heart.

When I found situations confusing, I relied on him to listen to my problems and to express his opinions about them. Sometimes, when feeling timid, I just needed his encouragement to go forward. And sometimes I really wanted to have him do a reality check for me. I didn't necessarily do what he said, but I valued his judgment and knew that he was a good sounding board.

For a few months after Dad's stroke, we all operated under the same illusion that the physicians were surely wrong. There was a sense that we could get things under control. But over time, Dad's recovery was limited. His dementia only got worse. And we had a sense that he would die, the ongoing feeling that *this would be his last birthday. This would be his last anniversary. This might truly be the last visit.*

I realized that the part of him that was giving, gracious, encouraging, grateful, and kind was not housed in his mind. We still enjoyed this familiar part of his heart. And if, as he said, one looked at kindness as the measure of one's contribution to a meaningful life, then he continued to have a meaningful life.

One day only a month into his illness, he looked at Jan and me and said: "Someday I'll have a funeral, and at the funeral I want you to thank all these kind people who have taken such good care of me."

I remember smiling and thinking that I would be sure to do that. My smile also reflected my understanding that as he was receiving so much kindness, he wanted to make sure that he expressed his gratitude.

Dad's sense of appreciation and engagement with everyone working at the nursing home was one of the pluses. He might have been confused, but he was generally willing to listen and still curious about everyone "in the organization," as he said.

He made it a point to tell people that they were doing a good job. I once watched as a nurse dressed the leg wound that plagued him for many months. Dad complimented her expertise. He looked up at me and declared that she was just the best one at healing this problem. And he turned to her and said what a good job she was doing, as she applied the triple antibiotic ointment on a gauze pad and wrapped it around his leg.

He encouraged me to encourage others, too. When I told him about some books on tape I had borrowed from the library, he said:

"If it's good, why don't you send them a note telling them that they have a great voice?"

"Really?" I said. I had never written a note of appreciation like this. It felt extreme to me.

"Yes," he said firmly. "People need to be appreciated for what they do. It gives them a sense of pride." He then started to laugh. "I need it too."

◇

In Dad's world he didn't always know where he was. He wasn't sure what his purpose was or if he worked at the place where he was living. He felt responsible for everything going on around him.

He complained to me about the status of his roommate, saying that he was *meshuggenah* (Yiddish for "crazy"). Dad was upset, adding that he was responsible for his roommate. I sometimes wondered how he managed to become so responsible, but I imagined that it just happened one day that he saw that he had to take care of him and the kindness became another frustration. He didn't know that his deteriorated state was similar to that of his roommate.

◇

During one visit, Jan told Dad: "I hope that I can learn to be as kind as you are. I don't know how to do it."

In a fatherly mode, he advised, "You just have to see the part of the person that is really good. We all have that part in us. It takes another person to see it."

But Dad's roommate, who often troubled Dad, chose that moment to contribute to the conversation.

Dad replied: "Shut up, or I'll come over there and knock you out."

Jan trying to calm him down said: "Dad, what happened to being kind and seeing the good in everyone?"

Dad didn't miss a beat. He said: "I *am* being kind—by not killing him."

But typically Dad's kindness was of a more gentle variety. Dad had a value, an ideal of kindness that he tried to live. In this moment, when his ideal was something he could still talk of but could no longer embody, we his children had to now embody these values. He could no longer maintain them. But he was clear that this was what mattered to him, and he continued to do the best he could to be kind, generous, and grateful. He had set the example.

Chapter 12
Love is All Around

By June, it had been four months since Dad had his stroke. I called the nursing home daily and called my siblings every few days. I also reached out to friends and extended family seeking personal support. No matter what my plan was for the day, there was always the question mark of what unexpected needs demanded my full attention. I was in the question of my father's condition, all the time.

Dad was 90 years old. We had talked about death and his feelings about it all through the years. He wasn't afraid of death. He was sure that he wouldn't have a prolonged illness, he said; "after all, I'm already so old." I knew his opinions. We all did.

We all had to stay in the present and react to only what was true at this moment, for it seemed the doctors' initial dire predictions were not correct.

As Dad traveled through his dementia, he became his true heart. I thought back to 20 years earlier, when I had felt his true heart after his heart attack. It was the same heart. But his practical ways and personality could no longer hold back his truth.

Once when my sister Jan called Dad, she closed the conversation with her usual: "I love you, Daddy." He replied, "Well, it's all around. Just join in."

My sister was so moved; she repeated this story at a wedding reception and enchanted the guests with Dad's innocent perceptions.

Or, as he said to my mother and me about my brother-in-law, Alex, "You know, he is one of these people that the more time you spend with him, the more you love him. And I'm not kidding. It's really so."

Or, when sometimes I wondered if he were in a stupor and ungrounded, he said, "Never forget how much I love you. Never forget how much I love you."

And I'd say, "Don't worry, Dad, I won't forget. And don't you forget that I love you like the stars love the sky."

"Double that from me," he would reply.

One of my favorite interactions came during a phone call in March of 2004.

"Hi Dad. It's Eve."

"Eve, I was just talking to your father."

"No, Dad. *You're* my father."

He exclaimed, "Really? What wonderful news. And Jan?"

"She's your daughter, too."

"What a wonderful day. I'll be darned. Great news."

We continued our conversation, but I can't remember the topic. I found myself in wonder of how loving this man was in his innocence. Even if he was more and more disoriented, when he could, he received the descriptions of his life with a delight.

Maybe that was it. With this illness, Dad delighted in experiencing love. After all, he just needed to be reminded of the specifics of the relationship—he already felt the love.

Chapter 13
Humor

Dad was a thoughtful and responsible man. Even when I was a young child, whenever we spoke, he made me aware that life was serious. I always wanted to play, but that didn't ever seem to be his interest. From him, I observed how being responsible was important. I often remember feeling on guard in his presence and needing to watch my behavior. I didn't want to do anything to make him unhappy or mad. He was the serious parent. He stood with his arms folded against his waist. It made him seem so formidable. So when he did things that were unexpected, I was shocked and amazed.

Yet for our whole family, our most common defense mechanism was humor. When we were happy or when we were sad, jokes served us. We each had our own type of humor. Mom was a performer and had a slapstick quality. Craig's humor was on par with any standup comic. I was sarcastic and always laughed the loudest. Jan was quick and original.

Dad's jokes were always clever and surprising. This very serious man delighted in setting the world upside down, just for a moment in time. He enjoyed telling long stories in which he convinced someone that something totally outlandish was true. He even made up new words for common things in the stories.

When I was a little girl, my father brought bagels when he picked up my sister and me at Sunday school. Partially he would do this to satisfy any immediate hunger, but I think it was also to prevent us from getting carsick. He always began our ritual the same way, saying, "Now, you girls have to remember to eat the bagel holes. You keep leaving them in the car, and your mother gets so mad at me."

I remember laughing with great delight as I took my fantasy bite into the imaginary bagel holes, reporting when they disappeared, participating in the conspiracy to appease the imaginary complaints.

It was a long ride home, so to amuse us he told stories about a character named Backwards Joe, who thought he was supposed to do the exact opposite of what he was told. If that didn't keep us in giggles, he could always fall back on the one song that I remember him singing: *There's a Hole in the Bottom of the Sea*.

Dad reported that during one of his buying trips to New York City, he went to a drugstore counter and ordered a scoop of vanilla ice cream. Then he asked for mustard and ketchup. He proceeded to pour the condiments on the ice cream.

The waitress asked, "Are you going to eat that?"

He responded, "No, but isn't it pretty?"

He stared at it for a several minutes, paid the bill and left. I was about 10, and I thought he was not capable of such absurdity. And I was amazed that the straight man in the story was his waitress. He was totally engaged.

◇

The rich, self-effacing quality to his humor remained.

When he was about 85—before any strokes or dementia—he told my brother Craig: "You know, most of my friends are dead. When I die, to get anyone to come to the funeral, you are going to have to make an offer of a funeral with free movie tickets."

One day when I went to visit Dad, in the summer of 2003, he told me he had some bad news.

"Oh, really? What is your news?"

"Well, I've been fired from my job."

"Oh, no, Dad. I'm so sorry."

"Yes. But I wasn't able to do a good job anymore. After all, I am 70 years old."

I said, "Dad, dearest, you are 90 years old."

"Ninety years old and I had that job? No wonder they fired me." Then he caught himself and found himself remembering his age—and at that moment, he started to laugh.

Another time, later that year, I phoned Dad with some less-than-good news: I had broken three bones in my foot and was wearing a huge purple cast. He was very sympathetic. Then he warned: "You've got to stop all that jitterbugging."

I wanted to know how his day was going. So I asked him if he had eaten breakfast, and he replied enthusiastically: "Yes, it's what lets me know that I've made it through another night."

A month later, on a bright, sunny November day, I called Dad and talked as I watched my dog play in the park. He asked me what was new, and I told him about my work.

He responded, "I want to quit my current job and get a new job, like working for you. But I need a good job title."

I said, "Well, I would be president of Sacred Intuitive Healing, and you can be the assistant to the president."

"I like that," he said. "It's not bad for a 91-year-old."

I responded: "But Dad, you're only 90."

"No, I turned 91 yesterday."

"No, Dad, it's November, the month of Jan's birthday, not yours."

He said, "No, my birthday is May 6th, and it was yesterday."

I gave up. What good was it doing to argue with him? It took all my energy to tell him I was right. What difference did it make anyway?

"Happy birthday, Dad," I said. "I'm so sorry that I forgot to send you a card."

He howled. I couldn't believe it. I said: "Well, aren't you a coyote?"

And he started to laugh harder. He had really gotten me.

Every person has a different tolerance for the kinds of omissions and memory lapses they can accept from a person with dementia. My brother told me that for him it was when Dad no longer remembered his name and called him Oscar, my uncle's name. Craig reminded or corrected him, saying, "I am your son, Craig." Dad would sometimes turn to me and ask, "When did Oscar change his name to Craig?"

On one visit in August 2004, Craig found Dad in his wheelchair in the common room, talking with an aide. Dad turned to her and said,

"This is my son, Craig."

Then he turned to my brother and asked, "How do you like that, Oscar?"

Staff members shared stories of Dad's humor as well. One staff member told me of a day in July, when a musician was strolling down the hall, playing a guitar and singing Christmas carols.

One of the other residents protested that it was summer, and therefore way too early for Christmas music.

My father had looked as if he were dozing. But he spoke up, saying: "It's never too early for Christmas."

Even in his dementia he was the ultimate retailer.

When I told Dad that I was writing a book about him, he looked surprised. He sat straight up in his chair, laughed, looked me in the eyes and said: "I hope it's interesting."

Chapter 14
Glimpsing Chaos

Many days, Dad woke up and found himself somewhere in the 1960s or '70s, not in the memory unit of a nursing home, but working in a large department store, with responsibilities for the merchandise. I would find him going through his closets as if he were going through a sales rack. He made notations on the frame of the closet. I couldn't make any sense of it. I assumed that he accounted for the inventory and was making plans for the coming week.

"Eve, I made a special purchase of some dresses on the 8th floor," he might say. "I got them for $100, and they are great. Let's go and let you try on some of them."

"You know what Dad, it sounds great. But how about I take you out, and we get some coffee?"

This became the run-of-the-mill confusion: He wakes up, finds himself somewhere, devises his purpose and what his role is, determines what his responsibilities might be, and goes forward. Other times, his lack of grounding produced a more disturbing interaction.

Once he spoke as if we were part of a magical fairy tale: "Eve, it's great you are here. But you are a princess and have to wait for the other princess and beware the queen." He went on and on about this kingdom that we were in and advised me to be careful.

These moments were more difficult, for they had no relationship to his past nor to a past I understood. If I tried, I could imagine that it contained a mythic quality, as do all fairy tales uncovering the human condition through their journey into the deeper recesses of the mind. But within these moments, I lost my Dad and felt myself interacting in a void where the mind had no past and had no future, and I was enmeshed within his journey of interpreting chaos.

In August 2003, I drove from California to Orlando, the highway taking me right by Dad's nursing home. It was a very rainy afternoon, and it was cool enough to leave my well-trained German Shepherd in the car, so I stopped to say a quick hello to Dad.

I lowered the windows just for a minute, sighed that my adventure driving across the United States was over, and breathed the fresh wet air. I let the dog out to visit the grass quickly and urged her back inside the car.

The nursing home was familiar now. I headed to the wing where Dad lived. Several staff people welcomed me back. They told me Dad was waiting for me.

I found him in his room talking with an aide and the nurse. They all turned to see his reaction at seeing me.

"Oh, Eve, you're so beautiful," he said. "It doesn't matter that you are black."

Okay. This was more than surprising. He couldn't see me. I had anticipated that there may come a time that he would not recognize me, but having it actually happen left me feeling a quick disappointment. He did not see what is there. He did not see me as who I am.

Remembering that I had committed to non-attachment to these changes, I said: "Thanks, Dad. I'm glad it doesn't bother you." And I went over and gave him a hug.

The next day I was sitting with him in his room while an aide changed the sheets. She was Haitian by background, and friendly and kind.

Dad asked her, "So, do you have brothers and sisters?"

"Yes, I do. Six. I lost one brother."

"I'm sorry," he said.

"Do you have children?" he asked her.

"Yes, I have two."

"How wonderful. How old are they?"

She answered, "Eleven and fifteen."

"Wonderful. I'd like to know more about your culture. You know, I have three great-grandchildren. They're white. I'd be happy to have some black great-grandchildren. I'd like some."

Somewhat in awe of my father's enthusiasm for more great-grandchildren representing the colors of the rainbow, I piped into the conversation with a mild amount of curiosity, "Dad, how would you do that?"

He stared at me in wonder at my question, and replied: "The post office."

"Okay, Dad. Let's keep our hopes up that you will have more great-grandchildren."

He turned to me. "Eve, I don't understand why black people are becoming white and white people are becoming black. How is this happening?" He looked bewildered. The aide folding the sheets stared at us silently.

I was uncomfortable that he had put it to me in the form of a question. Dad wanted to figure out what he was experiencing. I didn't know what to say. I didn't know what question to ask to be comforting or discerning. What did I know? I knew that the people who tended him were all shades. I wanted to think that maybe he could no longer make separations that keep us apart. Maybe his heart could no longer translate what he saw. But what was happening in his heart and his brain was increasingly chaotic. It was larger than his not knowing where he was and being disoriented. He couldn't see what was there. His reality shifted into realms we no longer shared. Black became white. White became black. And I didn't have the answer to the question he asked, about how this was happening.

Usually his alternate realities seemed clear to him. Where had his consciousness now wandered, and what elements now made up his world? He knew that his was not the reality that he had shared with us in the past. Where would I find an explanation? Could I tell him that he was now seeing all the lifetimes that we have? I didn't know whether this could be true, but I liked the thought. Everything I considered led me back to the mystery of his bewilderment.

"Dad, I don't know."

He shook his head back and forth and said, "I just don't understand it. It's so strange."

It was strange, and I allowed it to be beyond our comprehension.

The next day we went to the dining room for lunch. As soon as had wheeled him in place at the table, he said he wanted to stand up for the president of the corporation who was coming to have lunch with him.

"Eve, I have to stand up. Untie me." He was wearing a light restraint to prevent falls.

"No, Dad, we are just here to eat."

He was disgusted. "Eve, you are so stubborn." I had been called stubborn by him all my life, so I could easily stop listening when he said this.

"Dad, you're stubborn too." I had hoped to get him to laugh, but he was focused on the role he thought he was supposed to play with the president of the corporation coming in. I wondered what corporation he was thinking of, but I didn't ask.

He wouldn't eat his meal. One of the nurse's aides encouraged his belief in the meeting. She told him that it would be good to eat his meal first. I had no idea whether this was a good strategy or not. I found his frustration the hardest thing for me to deal with at this moment.

Finally, I untied the lap restraint. He stood up, balancing his hands on the top of the table. The room was nearly empty now. There were few people there and certainly too few to be called a meeting. But he started to speak. He was saying how important it was that we gathered to address the issues at hand. He didn't bring up an issue, though. He was trying to say something about what we were here for. How I wished that I could have given him the answer of why we were here and what we were working on.

Mostly he looked disappointed that he had messed up. He was irritated, frustrated, and angry. There was no way to guide him to focus on the possibilities in the moment, as he had created a moment when he had lost all possibilities.

We finished the meal. I took him to another part of the nursing home. I missed that our worlds so often didn't match. And I was sorry in this moment I couldn't help make anything better for him.

Chapter 15
Transfer

One thing the family learned from Dad's situation is to always expect the unexpected. For instance, here's an email I wrote in September 2003, about seven months after the stroke. It's one of many Jan, Craig, and I sent around to update each other:

Thought I would share what Dad said to me on the phone a little while ago. He was concerned with how things are going and that he wouldn't die well. I assured him that he was going to have an absolutely beautiful death. He seemed quite happy with this. It took a little convincing.

Then he asked me if the rumors were true about me. "What rumors?" I innocently asked.

He said, "That you are pregnant."

I told him unequivocally that I knew that rumor to be 100 percent false.

He said, "Thank God. It would be like it was from a virgin."

I said, "Dad, I'm not a virgin, but it would be similar in other ways. It would be like Sarah and Abraham in the Bible. I'm too old. It would take an act of God."

Life was always interesting with him, but I thought perhaps things were settling down some. We had our conversations and I cleared up confusion when it was possible, made regular visits, and tried to stay on top of his needs and the gradual progression of the dementia.

Then the wind was knocked out of me again. Days after I wrote that email, Dad was roaming in the nursing home and rummaging through someone else's drawers. When the other resident came over and tried to stop him, he slapped her hand four times. The facility informed us, as they always did after any incident happened. I could never get used to such episodes happening.

The next day the staff called Craig in to say that they thought an Alzheimer's facility was the best situation for Dad. The nursing home had to think of the well-being of the other residents.

Dad had been there for seven months, and I had finally come to terms with the idea that this was probably the best place for him. And now it wasn't. This is the way life is. Situations change. But the broader change can be where your parent is and where they need to be. And the most significant change was who he had become.

In the meantime, until we could find a new facility, I was afraid they would give him drugs to settle him down. They put him in what is called a Geri chair, which unlike a wheelchair, does not allow mobility. We were all concerned about the effects on Dad of being in a Geri chair. Would he get weaker? Would it be frustrating? Would he become angrier? One of the pluses of being in a large facility was that he could wander the halls. Even though he sometimes thought he was in an airport, a jail, or a hotel, he had mobility, and he was the one who identified exactly where he was.

You might imagine that when a person awakens each day believing he is in a different environment that one more change of place won't make a difference. Unfortunately, that is not the case with people with dementia and Alzheimer's. Even though Dad's world was unstable, it did generally have the stability of this nursing care facility. Making a change in location is a gigantic adjustment.

Within the same week, my own mobility took a hit: I fell down some stairs and broke a number of bones in my foot. I made some jokes about how people often mirror their animals, sharing the same symptoms. Now I was mirroring Dad's reality. It was trying and exhausting to move very far. It fell entirely to my brother, sister, and niece to research and select the new place and help with the transfer. I also identified with my father when he voiced the sentiment that he was not meeting his responsibilities to our family. I felt I was no longer able to be useful.

The universe wanted me to stay put, and having a cast on my leg was the ultimate test. The cast was on my left foot so at least I could still drive, but just walking around a grocery store with the cast was absolutely exhausting. I meditated, quieted, and made my world small for the time being. While the cast was on, I spent each day reading a book in bed. This was a significant change for me. I couldn't travel to Florida. I had to relax. It was what I needed at the moment, but the question—and the fear—was about how I could contribute.

After all these months, I finally understood that Dad would not return to being the person he had been. He was 90 years old and loved by many. Now the question was only where he would be happy. Just as he wanted that for me, I so wanted him to have happiness in his final days.

I looked to the Tao Te Ching for some sense of balance and harmony in this time of great transition. The Tao is a book that celebrates the process of change in one's life and the connection to the greater forces in the universe. As always, I opened the book hoping that whatever page I turned to would help me in this moment.

Chapter 13 (as translated by Stephen Mitchell)

Success is as dangerous as failure.
Hope is as hollow as fear.

What does it mean that success is as dangerous as failure?
Whether you go up the ladder or down it,

your position is shaky.
When you stand with your two feet on the ground,
you will always keep your balance.

What does it mean that hope is as hollow as fear?
Hope and fear are both phantoms
that arise from thinking of the self.
When we don't see the self as self,
what do we have to fear?

See the world as your self.
Have faith in the way things are.
Love the world as your self;
then you can care for all things.

I read this and felt the truth that all the worrying I was doing only kept me behind the potential of what might be possible. It only represented what I already knew, and not what I didn't know. It was time for a change. Maybe in an Alzheimer's facility, Dad would be happier. And maybe I needed to learn to release my adored sense of having some control over things, both my body and my family's well being, and learn the gentleness and tenderness toward all things, including myself.

We found a good place. Now Dad would live in a facility where everyone had a similar memory problem. There would no longer be room to take denial with me as my protection. And there would no longer be enough room to take the hand of fear and worry along the way. I would walk with tenderness and commit to be open to all possibilities.

Chapter 16
The Thanksgiving Visit

Dad's new home was a memory unit. We imagined that it would be a difficult adjustment period; the facility required that the family hire a professional sitter to be with him the first week. Jan, who had helped with the transfer, said the place was beautiful and that Dad seemed comfortable there. We were all amazed at how mobile Dad had become. He was no longer in a wheelchair, and no longer had restraints. He was free to use his walker anywhere around the facility.

In the other nursing home, he had nearly always been in a wheelchair, mostly with a lap restraint, because he was a fall risk. I had relied on the staff's assessment of Dad's state of being, not questioning this aspect of care. After all, they were always available for check-ins. During monthly meetings with the staff, they updated us about mental, emotional, and physical changes. I rested, knowing that the professional care was good and that he was loved.

I was worried that in the memory unit, he might not be as well loved and appreciated. Luckily, I was able to visit just a few weeks after the move, at Thanksgiving. We gathered as a family for another holiday and once again, I felt that the universe provided the opportunity for more time together.

Dad seemed in good humor in our phone conversations. Every day he packed all of his things, awaiting the "time to go." Everyone in the place spent a good deal of time packing, imagining they were leaving to go home to their families. Dad was up all night before I arrived, roaming the halls with another resident, looking for the train to New York.

When I walked into the memory care unit the day before Thanksgiving, I still had a boot cast on my injured leg. Dad looked down at my leg, concerned, startled, and upset. I told him that it was fine: "It's getting better everyday."

The memory unit facility was serene and lovely, with a courtyard with skylights, and real plants, and loveseat swings where you could sit and talk. There was room and freedom for Dad to roam.

I looked around at the other residents, whose expressions seemed far less lively than Dad's. It was frightening to imagine that Dad could become like that as well.

A leg wound that had bothered Dad since August still had not healed, and his diabetes was not yet under control. His feet were swollen, and his shoes weren't the right size anymore. Clearly, there were many problems to address during my visit.

Dad had his Army picture posted outside the door of his room to help identify the room. He showed me the picture, telling me "this picture can be found all over the store. Do you want a picture? I could get you one."

"No, thank you. I'm sure that I already have one."

He wanted to take the elevator to show me the rest of the place. Unfortunately, it was a one-floor facility. But I went with him, knowing that under the best of circumstances, he would be easily distracted from the need to find the elevators.

We ran across a cart with cleaning products, and Dad started to take some of the plastic gloves for me, just in case I wanted them. I said thanks, but really the staff needed them for their work.

He insisted he had the authority to get them for me.

I didn't want him to lose his authority over a plastic glove, so I said I'd take just one. I kept it in my belt.

The staff here didn't seem as friendly as in the other facility, but it was comfortable and homey. There were televisions on that no one seemed to be watching, and there was music playing in the background.

Because it was Thanksgiving week, it seemed that there were many other family members visiting.

My niece's in-laws held a Thanksgiving feast with almost 50 adults and about a dozen children. Dad loved looking around and seeing all of the children and smiling at the various adults. He remembered most of them. Everyone made a great deal of fuss about him. People were surprised to hear him making jokes.

He looked strong. At one point in the evening, I saw that he was alone at the table, eating a sugar-free dessert. I went over to him and said, "Dad, everyone is talking about how great you look."

"They should have seen me 50 years ago," he said.

We both started to laugh. We were able to have an almost-normal moment, in which we carried on in all the old ways. It had now been nine months since the stroke, and if anything, he was more independent, and stronger. He was clever and self-effacing as he had always been. I realized how much we underestimate the strength of the human spirit. To the people who hadn't seen him, he appeared much more in control of his senses than he was. If a person talked with him for two minutes, he seemed almost normal, but if they stayed by his side for some 10 minutes, he drifted into other realities readily and easily—telling you he was 70 years old and needed to get another job, or asking which holiday it was that we were gathering to celebrate.

I questioned, as all my family did, why and how he was able to be so much more ambulatory than he had been just a few weeks before. The truth is that he had many more falls. He was not absolutely steady on his feet. There was a trade-off here: his risks were greater, but so was his strength and independence. Being independent can be as simple as being able to use the toilet by oneself, or not needing personnel to support him for every activity.

The following day a friend and colleague of mine, Nicole, came to visit from Miami. My brother and mother had moved into a new apartment, and I was reluctant to offer her a place to stay prior to visiting their new place. But within five minutes, my mother invited her to spend the night. Wherever she and Dad called home, it always had a warm and open atmosphere where guests were welcomed.

The family invited us to join them at a movie, but Nicole and I decided to spend time together to talk and to visit with my dad.

When we got to the facility, we found Dad packing all his things into a large box. He told us that he was moving out soon, and he needed to get all his things together. In the past I had found it helpful to just let him pack and knew that the aides there would unpack his things later.

He was happy to meet Nicole, and within five minutes he suggested that she spend the night to take advantage of all the activities in the area. I was pleasantly surprised that my mother and father took about the same amount of time to invite another person into their circle.

We sat and talked. Dad showed Nicole the memory book containing his life story, which he could no longer tell. He was able to tell us that his granddaughter Laurie had put this book together, and he was proud.

But I noticed that he didn't have his dentures in, and I couldn't find them in the bathroom. I left Nicole with Dad and went to find an aide to see if they might be more successful than I had been.

The nurse found me searching for an aide and she and an aide came into the room to help with the search. They wondered, as I had, whether he had thrown his dentures away in the trash that had already been picked up for the day. Maybe Dad had packed them. We looked through all his things with the end conclusion that if they were gone there was nothing that we could do now.

Losing things and finding things and assuming ownership of other things were just par for the course at this point. I just hoped that he had stashed them away for safekeeping and that they would show up.

I joined Nicole and Dad in conversation. Dad was asking her how she knew me and she was explaining that we met years before, when I taught at the acupuncture school she attended.

He started to focus on me and said, with regret, that if he had had more money, I could have had greater educational opportunities, and

I would be a professor.

"What do you mean?" I asked.

"Well, if you had gone to a good school, you could teach in a university."

"But Dad, I went to a good school. I went to graduate school at Columbia University."

"You did?" It was clear that this was news to him. "Well, you could have gone to a better school than that."

"I don't know. But it's okay. I do teach; I teach acupuncture."

"Still, you should have gotten more and a better education." Dad had taken a position and it was final. Dad always held fast to the belief that education was the key to success. He regretted that in the late 1930s, he didn't have the $25 to pay for his next semester at Toledo University to continue his education. Now he was in a place of regrets, and he regretted what he thought he hadn't done for me. It was so personal for me that I engaged completely in the discussion, defending myself, and my life.

Realizing that we were at a stalemate, Nicole said: "You are very proud of her, aren't you?"

I remember thinking that Nicole's timing was impeccable, and I was grateful that she was there to stop me from arguing.

With tears in his eyes and a voice that was breaking, Dad said, "Yes, very proud. And she went through so much during the Depression."

Nicole and I looked at each other. Suddenly both of us felt our eyes fill with tears, realizing that Dad was emotional and vulnerable. He was recounting other events in his life that must have had to do with a sister, or mother, or perhaps all the women in his family, who were now somehow blended together. Clearly, it didn't have anything to do with me. He had regrets, but they were the generic kind—that he hadn't done enough. It didn't really matter whether he spoke of me, or his sister, my mother, or his grandchild. He just needed to say that he wished that he had done more for us than he did. I felt the sentiment, and I left, giving him a kiss with a slightly saddened heart. I wondered if he would learn to let go of his own judgment.

I said: "Let me put your mind at ease. You are a great dad."

At times I felt that I didn't know this man, because he was so humble and never told me stories that made him shine or sounded boastful. Nevertheless, no matter what, this man stood beside his family. Even in this moment, when he wasn't sure which member of his family I was and what our history was, he stood with me.

I didn't have to acknowledge his feelings, but I had to acknowledge the connection that he cherished. He was maintaining his heart and his presence in all our lives. He was still grappling with the issues that had occupied his mind for decades. He continued forward. He would have another opportunity to resolve these issues. We would remind him of the role he played in our lives. No matter what, he was still becoming more. He was resolving his ongoing issues, where the challenge was whether he had done enough in his life, and the impact was that in releasing some of these regrets, he was becoming closer to his truer self.

Chapter 17
I Don't Want to Be in the Army Anymore

While the memory unit was working out well, this didn't mean making the many day-to-day decisions got any easier. Often, I wondered if we could take care of Dad on our own. Insurance wasn't paying for any of his care. His retirement fund was dwindling, as monthly bills could go as high as $5,000. And there were ever increasing expenses to take care of my mom, as well. This was not the reality that Dad would have anticipated in his wildest dreams. Several years before this, I brought up the subject of long-term health care insurance, and he said he was sure that he wouldn't need it. Now, with his prolonged illness requiring special care, we needed to rethink long-term care for both my mother and father.

But just when I thought it might be possible for us to care for Dad, he faced a physical or other challenge that would show me he needed monitoring we couldn't provide.

Dad had been receiving his medical care through the Veteran's Administration. When I visited in January 2004, the nurse at the memory unit shared concerns about Dad's fluids and the swelling in his leg. So we made an appointment at the Veteran's Administration clinic.

Craig and I discussed whether I could take Dad to his appointment on my own, but I was so unfamiliar with Orlando's roads that we decided to go together.

Dad's appointment was about an hour after lunch—so we didn't have to worry about his sugar levels. We wheeled him out to the car and got him situated.

Within a few minutes he began asking, "Where are we going?"

The first time he asked, Craig gently and succinctly answered that we were going to the Veteran's Administration to see the doctor and get some medication.

He turned to Craig and asked, "Did you know my daughter is in town?"

And Craig said, "Yes, she's in the back seat."

"Hi, Dad. I'm sitting behind you."

"Oh," he said. That was the end of his news.

After a few more minutes he asked again, "Where are we going?"

With an increased level of frustration in his voice, my brother repeated that we were going to the VA for a doctor's appointment.

"Is there a bathroom there?"

Craig, alarmed, turned to him and said, "Yes, but it's just 10 minutes away. Can you wait until we get there?"

Dad said he could, while I wondered if I would need to take him to the bathroom in the Hardees up the street. Then Dad asked again, "Where are we going?"

I thought Craig would be insane soon. I wondered why Dad never acted this way with me. How much is volition? I took him out often enough for coffee and burgers, so why was he less agitated on those trips?

But we made it there. I found a wheelchair, and then Craig took Dad into the clinic while I parked the car. First stop would be the bathroom.

I waited for them outside the men's room. Craig came out and asked if I would get an orderly. Dad had diarrhea.

I looked around at this place, a huge medical office building with a good deal of outpatient services. I went up to one desk, and they referred me to another desk. I went to another desk, and they referred me to a nurse's office.

There I explained that my 90-year-old father was in the bathroom with diarrhea and my job was to get whatever help I could. The nurse was sarcastic, asking why we had brought my father here.

I explained that he was a veteran and received his medical care here. I said again that he needed help.

She remained unsympathetic, and I wished that I didn't need her help. She handed me a couple of towels, and I went back to the bathroom.

Without much hesitation, I walked into the bathroom. My brother was standing over the bathroom sink, trying to rinse out my father's pants, that were literally full of shit. When my father saw me he started to get up off the toilet.

"Don't get up, Dad. It's okay."

Craig asked, "Did you get an orderly?

I told him that there were no orderlies to get, but I had gotten these towels and had enlisted the aid of a nurse if we needed help.

Meanwhile, men were walking into the bathroom. I told them to use a stall, because we were dealing with an emergency. They didn't seem comfortable, but I was not going to let gender differences stop me from helping my brother and father.

The situation for my father was terrible. I noticed that he had brown liquid on his hands, in his shoes and socks, and on the edge of his sweater. I started to untie his white shoes when I thought, *what am I doing? I'm going to take all these things off with nothing to put back on him.* He basically needed a new set of clothes.

I told Craig I was off to get more supplies.

Swallowing my pride I went back to see the sarcastic nurse. Luckily, this time there was another nurse who was more sympathetic.

I explained that I needed some plastic bags for all of Dad's soiled clothing, and I needed scrubs for him to wear. The helpful nurse went for the scrubs and I took plastic bags, rubber gloves, and more towels back to the bathroom.

I thought that we had planned ahead when we brought an extra diaper with us, but I had no idea how one could possibly prepare for a situation like this.

Armed with bags and more towels and gloves, I continued the work that my brother was already doing. Pretty soon, Dad was looking much cleaner, and I went out again to get the scrubs, thanking the nurse for her kindness.

I gave Craig the clean scrubs and took the soiled clothes to put in the car trunk. I left the VA men's bathroom, hoping never to be there again.

We actually made it on time for his appointment with the doctor upstairs.

In the waiting room, I sat quietly next to Dad, holding his hand. I wanted him not to feel at all bad about the earlier mess. Dad had always been a neat, meticulous person. We sat quietly for 10 minutes while Craig, ever an extrovert, talked with other people waiting.

After a while, Dad laughed and turned to me.

"What is it?" I asked.

"You had to come here to wipe the crap off your father." And he laughed. I laughed, too, feeling amazed at his good humor, while I worried that he would feel humiliated. I wondered if there was crap between us that we dusted off, and I also wondered if he had just been carrying a load of crap for years and years. I did understand that somehow he felt okay and not humiliated. He was able to have insight in this moment. I was happy if there was less "crap" on the physical, emotional, or spiritual level that he or I were burdened by.

He then said, "I'm really glad your mother wasn't here."

And I didn't ask him why, knowing that he would have found it more difficult to be okay if she were around. Somehow he had surrendered to what was happening to him.

Dad was the last patient of the day. Craig and I accompanied him into the doctor's office. The doctor, a man of about 60, continued to sit behind his desk when we walked in and hardly lifted up his head. He looked at Dad's chart and began talking mostly with my brother. Craig explained that the nurse at the memory unit had requested that we bring Dad in to have his leg wound and swelling addressed.

The doctor took a cursory look. He said that Dad had to keep off his feet, keep his legs raised, and follow a salt-free diet.

We explained that Dad had extreme diarrhea on the way over, which was why he was now in scrubs.

Dad had a look of bewilderment on his face. He was quiet and looking from one person to the other. He didn't have the composure and insight that he had had in the waiting room just a few minutes before. He looked like he wanted to participate, but he couldn't get the drift of the conversation.

The doctor walked over and asked Dad whether the leg was causing him problems. Dad didn't seem able to respond right away. I was there holding his arm though trying not to be in the doctor's way. I saw that Dad looked tired. I wondered if he was sick and dehydrated.

I asked specifically if we needed to do something for Dad's immediate problem of diarrhea. The doctor said to just change his diet. I thought, *I need not have asked*. But the doctor seemed unconcerned.

As the conversation wasn't directed toward Dad, the effect was that it was more disorienting for him.

A doctor from the VA wound clinic came in and dressed Dad's wound. No change was made in his medications. We spent time in the pharmacy waiting to refill his current prescriptions. Dad fell asleep during the long wait.

It had been five hours since we started out. I was tired, and couldn't stop wondering how to best take care of Dad. A part of me wanted to kidnap him and take him away.

On the way home Dad was not the talkative man that he had been on the way there. He was exhausted. I called ahead to the memory unit to let them know that Dad had diarrhea and that he needed a special diet.

I spoke with one of the staff nurses who immediately told me that he needed doctor's orders to have his diet changed. I had reached my breaking point.

"What kind of doctor's orders do you require to know it is necessary to give a person toast, liquids, rice, and bananas when they have had diarrhea? I ask you. Is this reasonable?"

"I'm just telling you what is needed."

What could I do? She was just following procedure.

While my brother was gassing up the car, I went into the 7-Eleven and got bananas and water. When I got back in the car, I immediately handed these over to Dad, as if I were providing much-needed medicine. We stopped and got some white rice at a Chinese restaurant, and ordered some soup for Dad. We got back to the facility and got him situated at the dining table, and then left, exhausted.

"I'm really glad I didn't send you there on your own, given what happened," Craig said.

I was glad that there was more than one of us to do a three-person job.

The next day I arrived at the facility after breakfast. I didn't see Dad in the common area. I headed to his room.

He was lying on his roommate's bed, looking at the ceiling.

"Oh, Eve, I'm so glad to see you. We have to talk."

I sat down on the edge of the bed and took his hand. "What do we have to talk about?"

"Eve, I don't want to be in the Army anymore."

"That's okay, Dad. You don't have to."

"Eve," he looked at me directly in the eyes, "I'm not competent."

I couldn't help myself. Hearing his earnest self-assessment, and feeling my own grief about his situation, I started to cry. These were the tears that were always waiting to come out. These were the ones I held back all the time that came from some deep well inside me. They seemed endless.

Dad was digging into his pants pocket and he came out with a clean, folded napkin, which he put in my hand.

I remembered that Dad had always carried a clean, pressed handkerchief in his pocket. And though he might not be "competent," old habits die hard. His simply offering this napkin gave him another opportunity to remain my father who still comforted me, even as he accepted that he could no longer be the man he once was.

Chapter 18
Coming to Clarity

I spent some of that June in 2004 in a workshop in Montana, far from phone access. It was both startling and good to be out of touch. For the past year, I had been so entwined in the reflections that began with my father. Here, I was in a much-needed moment of pure self-reflection.

Yet what was most striking to me was how much I had missed being in contact. I called on Father's Day, as I drove home to California from Montana. Dad was excited: Craig was about to pick him up for a Father's Day celebration. He would see his great-grandchildren and Laurie. He spoke again of how he read the memory book she had made him every day. Even if he didn't really read it every day, it was a point of reference that he could always look at, and it was short enough to keep his attention.

He asked me what was new, and I replied that I was in Idaho driving home from a workshop in Montana. I told him about seeing antelope, elk, bear poop, and riding horses. I was in total awe of the landscape. He replied that it was wonderful to live a life where you travel and explore other countries. And he told me how proud he was of me. His ease in expressing affection was increasing with each month.

By the next day, he was totally different. He cried on the phone, saying he wasn't much of a man, with only two dollars in his pocket from his birthday. I tried to distract him, asking about the Father's Day celebration and the great-grandchildren. He said it was wonderful, and they were wonderful. But he was so upset he couldn't be distracted. He said he felt misunderstood and had no one to talk to about it.

"Wait, Dad. You have me," I replied. "You can talk to me. We are talking about it, and it's fine."

He said, "I shouldn't be talking to you. It isn't your problem."

"If it's your problem it is all of our problem. So it is fine and it will be okay. It is fine to express your frustration. Is that what you feel?"

And then he took off on another tack: Where was he going to go? How was he going to leave this place? Maybe Toledo would be better.

The next day when I phoned, I braced myself for more agitation.

I told him that I was just back from Montana, and he asked if I did any business. "Yes, Dad I went there for business," I answered. He laughed, recognizing my familiar sarcastic tone.

He started to talk about his brother, who was almost 97. "And he is as capable as anyone. He's going to make it to 100, and he deserves it. His wife is taking such good care of him."

Should I say it? I asked myself whether was kind to correct him still. "No, Daddy, it's his daughter, Lois, who is taking care of him."

I said it. He didn't take it as a correction; he was fine.

He said, "She's a nice person."

Then he told me that he would give me his address shortly, after he moved.

He told me that he loves me more each day. And the days are longer in the summer. And he was going to take advantage of each day.

"What will you do?" I asked, loving his hopeful tone.

"Enjoy it."

What more could I hope for?

"Craig's wife is recovering," he said.

"You mean your wife?" I asked.

"Well, I get no benefit. As the days go by we are building for new people who are joining our party." He continued the conversation from his own world.

"What party is this?" I asked.

"Well, everyone is making it to 100. I want the good grades. The only book written for us is Laurie's. I talked with Laurie to do something to expand that group. She seemed favorable to do it that way."

He paused. "Listen, I don't want you to spend all your money on this call. Best of luck and happiness. Thank you for calling. And your name is?"

"Eve, Dad my name is Eve. Who am I?"

"Aren't you that snobby little girl in California?" And he started to laugh.

He pondered, "Let's see, who are you married to?"

I replied, "I'm not married, Dad."

He was aghast. "Oh, that's horrible."

And then he retreated. "Listen, I'm 91 years old, and I haven't had a sweetheart in 60 years."

"No, Dad, you've been married for 60 years."

"Well, I didn't get much from it. I have handled it okay. I'm not greedy. She was a nice girl. I really didn't understand her. Listen, I'll tell Mom you called."

"Okay, Dad. Remember, I love you like the stars love the sky."

By the end, we were clear. I was his daughter he loved more each day. He wanted to enjoy each day. He is married and doesn't understand why he feels disconnected, though he admits he never understood her. This was absolutely true. And lastly, he would let Mom know I called, so he felt connected again.

And I wondered what would tomorrow be like in his world. If it was up and down for me, how must the world appear to him in his confusion? But then again, he still sometimes found clarity around what remained, what he couldn't be confused about.

Chapter 19
Deteriorating

I wasn't looking forward to returning to Florida in August, the hottest and most humid time of the year. But I felt I had to go, because the medical staff at the memory unit where Dad had been for almost a year said he was deteriorating. I hadn't noticed any difference on the phone, but my sister noticed a change when she visited a few weeks before. I wanted to spend as much time as I could while we could still laugh together and maintain familiarity. I had no sense of his spirit weakening, so I was going without fear about his physical condition, just his mental deterioration.

I called in July, shortly before I left.

"Evie, where are you?"

"California."

"Are you arriving tomorrow?"

"No, Dad, it's Sunday. I arrive on Friday night, but I won't see you until Saturday. I arrive at midnight."

"And Jan, when does she get in?"

"Well, Dad, she isn't coming this trip. You just get me."

"Okay, then. Well, I have good news."

"Yes?"

"I found you a great hotel room with a double bed and a single bed. And it's for free. It will save you money for the trip."

"Great, Dad, I look forward to it."

I thought that the room must be at the memory unit, and I would take a rain check. I noted that Dad still was the one in charge of finding suitable accommodations. He was the organizer for all family events. And he still was anxious to do that job.

As promised, after arriving on Friday night, I went to the memory unit at 11 the next morning. I looked across the common area to see if Dad was participating in some type of activity and then went to his room, where he dozed in his armchair.

I put my hand on his arm, and he opened his eyes slightly. After a couple of nudges he really opened his eyes and saw me there.

"Evie, oh, you're here. How was your flight?"

"I'm fine. I'm tired, though. I got in very late last night."

He started to tell me about not falling asleep until 4 a.m.; that Craig had been over the night before and had explained a project he was working on. At the end of the sentence he had fallen asleep again. I shook him a little, and he continued on, then started to fall asleep at the end of his sentence. I decided to check his blood sugar levels with his nurse. Sometimes I had missed that Dad was suffering from low sugar, thinking he was just tired, and then he would end up in an emergency room.

His nurse assured me that his sugar was okay, adding "He was just was so agitated yesterday that they had to call Craig to come over to calm him down. He has worn himself out."

She reported that he had been calling her a liar and saying that he didn't believe anything that she said anymore, and he was ready to quit this place and wanted to go. She said that he was impossible to distract.

On the one hand I was thrilled that it wasn't an insulin reaction, and on the other hand I wondered about his agitation. Maybe he was just tired of being here.

When I went back to the room, Dad was speaking with an aide. Dad told me about his talk with Craig and how proud he was of him. He received a call from his 97-year-old brother and had a very normal conversation with him for about 15 minutes.

We then walked to the common area and Dad asked me: "What are all these white-haired people doing here?"

I explained that they all had a similar kind of memory problem that he had. We walked around the facility as the aides gathered residents for lunch. One aide was pushing a Geri chair for a more sedentary resident, clearly distressed, asking: "Where are you taking me? Where are we? What city is this?"

The aide took her time to consider an answer, and I heard Dad loudly respond, "Chicago."

At that point the aide said: "Reuben," with a certain reprimanding but indulgent tone.

I started to chuckle despite my best effort to ignore the comment, and then I turned to Dad and asked, "Do you think you are in Chicago?"

He said, "No, but he doesn't know."

I started to laugh. We had a little conspiracy that was fun, even if it wasn't nice. I loved that he could still make a joke. He couldn't be deteriorating so badly if the world could still be amusing to him.

He sat down to eat. I thought that was enough for this visit and left.

The next day Craig, Dad, and I went to a local deli, where we ordered Dad one of his favorite meals. Craig shared an email from a close childhood friend including photos from Detroit from when Craig was a child. I couldn't tell whether Dad actually recalled the places, but I think that he definitely enjoyed the sense of reminiscing with his son.

Craig wanted to surprise him with a quick trip to Laurie's house after lunch. We were on the road to her house when we heard him say, "This is the way to Laurie's house."

Both Craig and I were surprised. Whenever something like this happened, I always wondered what he could recognize and know. And then I wondered what he could learn.

When we made the turn to Laurie's street, he explained in some shock, "Are we going to Laurie's?"

Craig gleefully answered: "Yes!"

Dad was really excited to be at Laurie's. He loved smiling at the children. And they liked pushing him in his wheelchair.

Meanwhile, he started rambling about how he and his Army buddies used to tell the girls that they were in the Navy because the Navy guys shipped out for six months. He explained that if you didn't call them, it would mean that you had been shipped out. The rest of us laughed, thinking that this must have been some fantasy that he was experiencing. It's not as if a person couldn't tell the difference between Navy and Army uniforms. It must have been exciting for him to remember back to a far less limited reality.

He did have some cogent moments in the midst of his rambling. He said, "In my confused state, I'm really drawn to the periods when I was in the Army or working at the store. Those were really good times."

So we would bounce from one reality to another, never really understanding which part of what he was saying was true. But the sentiment of both enjoyment and sorting through the confusion was very real.

When I arrived the next day, Dad explained that he had had a big accident after breakfast and had had a bowel movement in his pants.

He said, "I was so embarrassed, the girl had to come to clean me up. Very few people saw me. It was okay. Thank God they do a good job helping me out here."

Just then the aide came in to check on him. She had been the one who cleaned him up.

Dad said, "I'm going to pay you next week. I promise."

She reassured him that actually it was all taken care of.

Then he started to talk about his R.J. Soldinger antique collection, worth thousands of dollars, that was at the estate. He really wanted to see it again.

In truth, Dad did collect antiques during World War II, but it hardly was enough for any exhibition. But these things remained important to Dad, and I think that he missed them. He also wanted to see his medals. I never remembered him looking at his medals, and I wondered where they were in the house.

I knew I couldn't give them to him. He couldn't hold onto his teeth most of the time. How could I bring him his medals?

I was thinking of giving him a clock CD player. I had tried giving him a CD Walkman last visit, but it had disappeared after several days.

He went for lunch and I left to buy a CD player, looking for the simplest one, with just an on/off button.

When I returned, Dad was in the hall near the entrance, having his sugar level checked. He was asking how long he had been there. He was looking around at everything as if this was the first time he had seen the facility. I told him he had been here a while, because he had a memory problem and medical problems and needed special care.

He asked me how much it cost a month. I told him it cost more than $5,000 a month. He was appalled that it was such a huge expense.

But then I changed the channel, so to speak, and we set up his clock/radio/CD player. Within no time we were in his room listening to music.

He said, "This is just great. I'm going to change my life to do things like this."

I was not sure what he was referring to, so I asked, "You like listening to music?"

"Yes. I have to learn how to do it."

I was encouraged and reviewed how to operate the CD player a few times. I didn't know whether he could do it right away, but he had learned to do so many things, and he had recognized the way to Laurie's the day before. I was hopeful that he would be able to learn this.

He talked about Jan, saying: "Well, she has a really good husband and a good job, salary, and she makes the best of things. You should find one like him."

"Well, you never know what might happen."

He said, "For me, either. Seems like the ones I'm interested in are married."

I didn't know whether or not to remind that he was married as well. But I thought, *what the hell.*

"Well, Dad, you are married too."

"No, we've been apart 30 years. I don't think I appealed to her."

"Why not?"

"I don't know. I wouldn't want to pass up any good-looking girl who was interested in having her way with me."

I wondered if he would feel less lonely if he were at home. He longed for a kind of intimacy that he thought he might never have.

The next day, Dad was a little more present and slightly stranger. I had to wait a while before being let in. Memory units are locked down so that the patients can't go wandering. From the outside, I saw Dad chatting with some of the other residents, looking at me and waving on the other side of the door.

As we walked to his room, three of the residents began to shout at each other, which made Dad begin to shout: "Stop this. Stop this right now. Let us through." One of the women decided to try to soothe Dad, as I imagine was part of her relationship with men in general. She kept telling him not to get himself worked up, and that it wasn't good for him.

I observed in amazement at this attachment she had to him, though I was pretty sure he didn't know her name. I saw how important being loved by a man still was for this woman, even if it wasn't one who she knew from her life.

We went to his room and I showed him again how to work the CD player and he was amazed at the sound again.

Then he told me that he had a story to tell me.

"Well, I am invited to what I believe will be business lunches which end up being just lunches. I swear to God, I finish lunch and take a bathroom break. When I return everyone is gone. It's really crazy. It keeps happening."

While time had become mysterious for him, at that moment time stood still for me too. I heard and understood that my father was experiencing his reality as if in a dream and asking me to help him to find the key. How could I help him sort it out? I felt myself pause as I gathered myself and let the information trickle through me. I didn't know what to do. No matter what, nothing was matching between what he thought and what was happening. This was now his world. And he was trying to share some of his experience.

Then he said, "And I have another problem. I'm worried about a lump I have in my 'private area.'" Here, I recognized my father, who would rather not say exactly what he was speaking of, not on this topic, not to his daughter.

It was alarming to find out this information, which he would have difficulty reporting to anyone. And I thought that there was no time like the present to get it checked. After all, it was much easier sorting all this reality than what he had been saying. I found the nurse and asked her. She had no idea a lump was bothering him and said she would try to get it cared for.

I went back to him and told him that I had talked to the nurse and she would give him an exam later. As I sat in his chair, I looked at the list on his night table. It listed the following items: haircut, tape to seal boxes, seal bags, groceries, razors, sunglasses, house slippers, and, last, but not least: small gun.

For as many years as I could remember, Dad kept a neat, prioritized list on his nightstand. This was familiar. But the last item on the list piqued my interest.

"So, Dad ... why do you want a gun? "

"Thievery," he replied matter-of-factly. "I have to do something about it. They take things all the time. It doesn't even have to be a real gun, but it would be good to be able to scare off these people."

I was pretty sure that Dad "acquired" things as often as anyone else there. "If it's before me, it must be mine" would be a fitting motto for most of the residents. But in this moment, Dad was reaching for justice. He would not tolerate thievery.

Then he asked me, "Eve, what would you do if you could do anything in the world?"

"I don't know, Dad. I don't think anything different from what I'm doing. I'm searching to find the right avenue of healing, and what will inspire me for the rest of my life. I think I would like to travel to Asia and see what they really do to heal people."

He responded with, "What did you have for breakfast?"

I couldn't dwell on the fact that we couldn't discuss hopes and dreams anymore. "I had a bagel."

"Is that all? I could get you some Jewish potato latkes. The chief cook and I are on very good terms."

"I'm glad to hear that you have friends here. But I'm just fine. The bagel was enough for me."

"I wish that I had told you earlier about my collection. It's beautiful. I have to see it first. If all goes well, I could have my Toledo friends put together a show. I might still be able to go there for a couple of days. I still have friends there. Strange, that once you have friends somewhere you have them in different places."

Just then a woman wandered into his room. I had often seen her around the facility. She was thin with black hair and had a vacant look in her eyes. But she always responded when I took her hand and asked how she was doing. She didn't seem quite as old as the other residents. I didn't think she was over 70 years old. Often when I saw her she was lying on one of the couches. She looked around at the walls and then wandered back out of the room.

"*Meshuggenah*," Dad said, using the Yiddish word for madness. "She's lost all her reasoning. She was a beautiful girl. She has been failing, like I have. She was a beautiful person. She came here just a few years ago."

Then it was time for us to look for the elevator, to get to the fourth floor of this one-story building. We stopped to talk with as many staff as had time to chat in the middle of the afternoon. We made a few jokes. People saw us having a pretty good time. I wondered how much longer we would be able to do this. And I understood that he was deteriorating. He could progress to just wandering from room to room, just like the woman who'd come in earlier. Even though he was mentally deteriorating, he was still observing the world and the people in it from a core place, even if he didn't understand everything that was happening.

Chapter 20
Finding What is Important

One of the mornings during this August visit I arrived at the facility as Dad was about to be served his breakfast. He sat at the same table for each meal with three other men. I brought another chair to this table for four and sat down. There was no conversation between the men. They did not have ongoing relationships, though they spent all their mealtimes together. They retreated in their mental confusion to their own joys and sadness. I didn't want to be a distraction from the focus they needed to finish a meal, but I thought I could ask questions and they could choose whether and how to respond.

I asked one of the men if he had seen his family lately. He told me stories about his son and his professional life. One man was looking at the newspaper. One man did respond in whole sentences, but he kept folding his napkin. But when I asked questions, they listened and spoke. Dad was always a great listener, and I saw that he too was paying careful attention.

After the meal, Dad and I returned to his room. I showed him one more time how to work the CD player. I always thought my Dad could do any task better than anyone else. I showed him how to use the start and stop buttons a couple of times hoping that he could do it. I thought it would be helpful to give him something to learn. I decided to put on a recording of Yiddish music.

He said, "Mother would have liked this."

"Oh, would she now?" I didn't know my paternal grandmother, so I didn't know this aspect of her. "She liked music?"

"Yes," he said.

"Do you mean my mother in the picture? She's a great singer."

He looked up at the large photograph of our family from the late 1960s on the wall and realized that he couldn't connect. He had trouble recognizing my mother. His eyebrows were furrowed as I kept trying to understand where to go in this conversation. Not knowing his relationship with my mother was more upsetting than not understanding how to work a CD player.

I said, "Dad, this is a picture of my Mom, your wife. Do you remember she was sick in the hospital in June with heart problems? She hasn't been well."

I could see that the confusion was upsetting him. I had gone past the point of clarifying reality, it hadn't worked, and I felt we both needed a major distraction. I suggested that he use the bathroom and that we take a ride to get a coffee and pick up a newspaper. Outings remained preferable to confusion.

We ended up at Starbucks. I stood in line beside Dad in the wheelchair. We got a few charitable looks from the other people in line, but I chose to ignore them and was glad that Dad didn't seem to be aware of the sympathy coming his way. Ten years before, when Dad could still pick me up at the airport, we always stopped at Dunkin' Donuts and sat at the counter, having the first check-in of our visit. I savored the time where he could act as my guide and make comments about how I was moving through my life. But our purpose on this outing was different than those check-ins. We could no longer have an intense discussion on world events, but we were there together as father and daughter, and being together was our communication.

I asked him if he wanted a *New York Times,* and he refused, saying that he preferred the local news. Classic Dad. I was relieved to find something consistent. I bought the *New York Times* for me, and an *Orlando Sentinel* for him. We got our drinks and sat down.

I started to read him the headlines from the *Times* as I might have a couple of years before. "Man in Custody Is Linked to 2001 Attacks," I read, and started to talk about the article. I looked up to see his face blank. He didn't recognize the subject matter.

I asked, "Do you remember the terrorist attack in New York on the

World Trade Center buildings? You know when the World Trade Centers came down?"

With clear eyes and consciousness, he looked at me and said that he didn't remember. I looked for a headline or information that he could let rise and fall in his memory. The grief of this event was not shared by him. In his world it never happened. There was no terrorist attack. There was no color code for perceived terrorist threat. And there was no fear. The stock market goes up and down and he can track that, but the events that in some ways have shaped our consciousness no longer shaped his.

I returned to the paper and looked for information about the stock market and job rates.

He did notice the details of his new surroundings. He noticed the product promotions in the Starbucks and recognized that he was in a different place and that the coffee was strong. I offered to get him some hot water added to it, but he declined the offer.

We were reading headlines in our separate papers, just as we had done for many years at the kitchen table. Soon I noticed that he had started to doze. It was time to return to the facility. I unlocked the wheelchair, and maneuvered it away from the table, toward the door. The door opened out, so I couldn't keep pushing him and still manage to hold the door from behind. Luckily I looked around and found one person who met my eyes and offered a hand.

We returned to the facility, and I left so he could take a nap.

After lunch I returned, bringing along my computer to show him pictures of a friend who had just had a child. He was engaged in seeing the beauty of this baby. Then he wanted to know the details about the computer. At times like these few minutes I could easily imagine that he could be faking the confusion the other 95 percent of the time. He remained interested in how things worked. He remained aware of sights and sounds around him.

He leaned back in his chair for a moment and then said: "I don't think I have long. I'm physically tired, and I'm 91 years old."

I was surprised. But it was an opening.

I asked, "What do you want to do? What is important to you now?"

"There's a long list of projects I want to do while I'm alive. I want to get my things in order ... like my antiques. It's an important part of me."

"And about you, I don't want a contrived marriage between you and another person," he added. I had no idea what he was referring to, except that he wanted me to experience true personal happiness and not any artificial substitute.

"Okay, Dad, I promise I'll go for love and happiness with a wonderful man."

"That's what I like to hear."

"Dad, you seem very tired."

"There's no reason. I had eight or 10 hours of sleep. The only thing I have that is negative is my tiredness."

It was time for me to leave and take a business call, so I excused myself, saying that I would come again.

Our conversation had been disjointed but very authentic about things in the world and how he saw himself. He still had things to look forward to. The time we had together had been beautiful. It was worth it for me, despite all the difficulties in finding one another in separate realities. I smiled with gratitude as I went to my car.

Chapter 21
Finding Truth

In that summer of 2004, I was living in Marin County, California, and traveling for work—to Tucson, Montana, Mexico, Paris, and Seattle. All the while, I felt the longing to be closer to my family. And the crises seemed to come one after another, like waves on the beach. Still, each of us stepped forward to meet each problem.

My mother was now on oxygen for her congestive heart failure. Visiting nurses, physical therapists, and aides were in and out of the house every day, to help her rehabilitation. Short walks exhausted her. She was able to do less and less for herself. As the health workers came less often, my brother's responsibilities increased. I could see his spirit was sinking. He told me he had been feeling lightheaded and was going to get a stress test.

I pointedly asked him how Dad was, assuming that he visited at least once a week. Increasingly, he replied that he hadn't seen Dad this week. The first time he said this, it was no big deal. Life is very busy when you care for two parents. But it happened more frequently, I asked why, and Craig answered, "I just can't see him like this anymore."

"I'm coming home," I said—making the decision in an instant. Craig had no idea that I meant coming to live in Florida. But I knew that he had shouldered the burden long enough, and that Dad needed care, attention, and connection—and so did Mom. It had been years since she had been able to do many tasks of daily living. I couldn't let my brother go under. The number of people needed to keep this family afloat was increasing. I needed to be closer.

So I packed up my apartment in a week's time, and made my way back east.

I arrived in Florida on November 20th, just as the roads in Florida were filling up with cars for the holidays.

My first stop was to see Dad. I got there as he was being wheeled down the hall by an aide. He was so happy to see me, reporting that he had just told an aide that he was waiting for me. Yet I found myself distracted by the number of bruises on his hands, and he had a strong smell of urine.

Then the aide came back with the towels.

"I was just going to get a shower. But I can do that later." He started to stand up politely.

I said, "No, you sit back down and get that shower."

"No, no," he said. "I can do it later."

"No, no," I said. "I think that you need to do it now."

"Why? Do I smell?"

I stood there wondering how not to hurt his feelings. How can I respect him as the parent and as a human being? I just had to be truthful here.

"Okay, Dad. Yes, you do."

"Okay," he said just as emphatically, but without embarrassment. We agreed I'd see him later.

So it began with twice-daily visits to cheer, love, accept, and orient my father.

I tried to help by bringing my mother to visit him. My second day home, I brought her in a wheelchair, with her oxygen tank in tow. I left her in a small family room near the entrance as I searched for Dad.

I followed the usual process, looking first in the common areas and then going to his room.

He was there, awake and lying in his bed.

"Hi, Dad. Mom is in the other room."

"Oh. Now that's a reason to get up," he said, as he sat up slowly.

I helped him put on his shoes and brought over the wheelchair, though he was already standing to walk to the other room. He always forgot that he now needed a wheelchair. I prompted him to have a seat in the wheelchair. I watched him sit up properly, to make a good impression.

As soon as we entered the room and saw Mom, Dad asked her how she was and how she was feeling. She had gotten out of her wheelchair and was waiting for us in a comfortable lounge chair.

She asked him in turn how he was.

He said he was good. But he mentioned that he was sick and tired of all the *shnorrers* here. I thought perhaps he meant the people who sleep on the couches—as in *schnoozing* away the hours in sleep.

"Am I missing something in this conversation?" I asked. "What are *shnorrers?* Are we talking about the people sleeping in the lounge chairs?"

"No," my mother said, "in Yiddish a *schnorrer* is a person who takes advantage or freeloads."

Dad continued, "There are a hell of a lot of them around here. And

I'll tell you I'm sick and tired of them. They are all over the place. And I don't get one red cent from them."

I thought perhaps he was kidding. His spirit seemed high and he wanted to be entertaining. It was a little unclear to me what he actually believed.

He looked around the room, remarking on all the "changes" in it. For us, the room was exactly as it had been. But not wanting to burst his bubble, Mom made mention of the lamp and a picture.

I asked: "Dad, what changes are you interested in making?"

He said: "I would put it on fire."

Mom and I laughed. Now we were sure that he was kidding. He was going to entertain us.

He continued, "I would torch the whole thing. I'd start from the bottom up. What floor are we on?"

"Dad, we are on the first floor."

And we asked him what floor he lived on, and he said the eighth.

He wanted to re-do the whole thing, he said, and he wanted to get rid of all the *shnorrers.*

Mom looked pale, and a little faded, I thought. She had laughed a bit, and there was more of Dad's personality showing than she had been used to seeing recently. I wondered why she couldn't make jokes back anymore. But I felt comforted that Dad had entertained us, and we had all enjoyed the company.

We were once again together over the Thanksgiving holidays. We brought Dad to the apartment that my brother and Mom now shared.

The apartment was new to him, but furnished with items from the house where he had lived before his illness. He looked a little uncomfortable finding himself here. He always spoke of wanting to be around his own things, but now that he was, I saw that it was all unfamiliar to him. His eyes couldn't take in the pictures and furniture that had always been a part of his life.

My brother called a number of friends and relatives and put Dad on the telephone. He was amazing. He wished people a Happy Thanksgiving and asked his standard "What's new?" He was able to have normal conversations, 10 minutes long. I was so impressed.

The day after the Thanksgiving weekend, things changed again. Sitting in his wheelchair near the door, Dad was looking at a newspaper. I came to his side, and he looked up and exclaimed:

"Evie. Oh, I'm so glad to see you. I feel so bad." He took my hand and kissed it.

"I feel so bad. I've been suicidal."

"Oh, Dad, why?"

"I'm so lonely. I'm sick." He looked me straight in the eye and shouted, "And don't tell me that I'm not. I can't keep doing this. And I was thinking about suicide. But how could I do that to my family? I love you guys, and I love Mother so much."

I put my arm around him and held him tight around the shoulders as he cried.

"I'm willing to cut my throat. But it would be a terrible thing to do to the family. Mother knows how I feel about her. I've trusted her more than any other human being. Your mother is wise. And smart, too."

"I hate feeling like a victim," he said emphatically.

And he cried harder.

He lowered his voice and slowly said, "Eve, it's such a horrible thing to think only of yourself. I hate being negative. I try to be positive about things and to look forward to the possibilities. But I am negative. I can't get myself on track."

"Okay. Dad. Things aren't easy. But they can be better or worse depending on how attached you are to each event. You are the person who has taught me that. It's how you treat a person that makes the biggest difference in life. So treat people well and we'll see what happens."

"The only person who believes in me is Irda."

Now I was confused. Who was Irda? I knew the names of most of the workers. But Dad was on a roll. My attempt to "redirect" his thoughts was feeble, and it couldn't ease his angst.

He knew he was truly confused. And he needed help and he hated that, hated himself, and what he saw as his shortcomings and disabilities. Dad had lived his life never wanting to be a burden. Once when he was still living independently with my mother, I suggested that maybe they could get some help from services like Meals on Wheels. And he rapidly suggested that that was okay for some people, but not them. He was 86.

Here we were, though, facing a reality where dependence defined his life.

All I could do for him was to embrace it all. Embrace the craziness, the loss, the heartbreaks, the confusion, and the underlying willingness to now, at this point in his life, expose it all.

I said, "Dad, I love you like the stars love the sky."

He said: "I double that."

◇

The following evening, as Craig, Mom, and I had dinner, Craig posed a question to me: "What was your most interesting case in your practice?"

Not to be evasive, but not thinking in those terms, I answered, "I don't know."

Mom said, "Oh, I know."

It was a little shocking to hear her answer for me, but I was curious. "What was it?" I asked.

She said, "Remember the time that the boy was drowning and everyone came to find you so that you could save him? And finally someone did, and you saved the boy's life."

I was stunned. Nothing like this had ever happened. I was already worn down from spending so much of the days with Dad in his illusions. It was a shock to hear that my mother now had a separate reality as well.

"Mom, I don't remember," I said. "Will you excuse me a minute?" And I went to the bathroom to be sick—and then give myself some time to collect myself.

When I came back they had finished dinner, and Craig was at the sink washing dishes. My mother retired to her room.

"Craig, that was shocking to hear Mom say that," I said.

"I'm glad you heard it," he said. "Things like this happen all the time. Do you know what she said when you went to the bathroom?"

"What?"

"She said: what's wrong with Eve, that she doesn't remember her own stories?"

I couldn't believe it—and yet I could. Mom was 84 years old. The statistics that I knew say that 50 percent of people over 85 have dementia. But both parents with dementia, at the same time? Granted, my mother's case would be considered mild compared to my Dad's, but still—this was now another reality to be figured into any possible life plan.

At least in my mother's delusions, I laughed to Craig, I was a hero.

I visited Dad every morning and evening. If I missed a visit, he would have extreme anxiety. Once a week, we went to brunch, somewhere that might be a little familiar and wheelchair accessible.

At first, the outings helped with his desire to leave the memory unit and go home. He was happy when he returned to the facility.

But I began to notice that he was becoming more anxious about going home for a visit. He didn't want to be wheeled around. His usual surroundings were already new to him much of the time. Taking him into another new surrounding was becoming overwhelming to him. I could see that fewer outings were ahead for us.

At one visit in early December, Dad suddenly turned to me and looked me straight in the eyes.

"Eve, I am so confused. Don't bother denying it."

I just nodded.

"Do you think that it would help to speak with a psychologist? Because I would. I swear to God, I would do whatever it takes."

"I don't know if it would help, Dad. Part of the problem is just plain age. And now you have this memory problem. But if you are interested in speaking to a psychologist I'll investigate the possibilities. I spoke with a psychiatrist from Germany who says that they do therapy for people with dementia there. Maybe there is something available here. I'll have to check on this for you."

"Eve, I swear to God, I'll do whatever it takes."

Chapter 22
The Fall

"Are you ready for some potato latkes?" Dad greeted me happily, when I picked him up to go to Laurie's house for the family Chanukah party. He had on a pale yellow jacket and some new pants. I told him that he looked quite dapper.

It was true. He really looked well. These family celebrations were so important for him.

Meanwhile, my brother was taking my mother; handling her took much more strength, because her ability to walk was limited. We needed to use two cars now, to handle the two wheelchairs.

The house was in pleasant chaos, with children running around and screaming with excitement. Craig's ex-wife and her parents were there, and gave familiar hellos to my parents. A large table in the kitchen held a menorah. Our arrival signaled the go-ahead to light the candles and begin the meal.

I was getting some food when my brother and I both turned and looked at Dad. He was playing with my mother's hair, with an intimacy that was sweet, natural, and loving. At this moment, he was not confused about who she was or what his relationship was to her. To my surprise, my mother responded by kissing him and touching his forehead with hers. I wanted them to have this private moment in this somewhat crazy time. I wished we could all vanish for a while. We sensed that any attention might interrupt them, so we all ignored them, in the same way that you look away when teenagers are flirting and kissing, and you don't want to interfere.

I liked having the independence to talk with everyone else there. Dad seemed to be enjoying the evening. I spoke with Laurie and Scott and played with the children. But a little while after I finished my potato latkes, I saw that Dad looked deeply sad—as if he might shortly burst into tears. I ran to him.

"Dad, what's wrong?"

He looked up, into my eyes and said, "I miss everyone."

I hesitated for a moment. Maybe I shouldn't say anything. He felt the loss and separateness of his life as he felt the connection with everyone in this evening. How do we remain connected, when our sense of increasing separation defines reality?

I said, "Every person here loves you and enjoys you. Take the opportunity to breathe it in."

He relaxed. He continued to make a connection. My own earlier ease and relaxation left, as now I needed to monitor his mood. I felt he was perceiving a new limit, and I didn't want to go beyond it. After a while, I thought that I noticed his anxiety rising again and decided to take him home.

On our drive back, I talked about the children, admiring how cooperative they were as they played.

Dad would respond by saying that they were all geniuses.

I thought: *He is okay.*

◇

Just a week later, I got a 3 a.m. phone call: Dad had fallen again. The memory unit was sending him to the emergency room.

He had already fallen once in the month since I had moved back to Florida, so I wasn't unduly alarmed. I anticipated what was ahead: answering questions from doctors, because Dad's information about himself was no longer reliable, especially when he was in unfamiliar surroundings.

I could see him on a stretcher from the other side of the ER glass doors. Sprigs of his white hair stood out from his head, and even from a distance I could see a bruise and some blood coloring the ring of his hairline on his balding head. The EMTs were standing by. I identified myself as his daughter, and they told me that he reported having hurt himself in a car accident. I laughed. He hadn't driven a car in many years.

I took his hand. "Hi, Dad."

"Evie!" He was wide-eyed with surprise at seeing me.

"Dad, you fell. How are you? I see you have a big bump on your head. Are you okay?"

Instead of answering, he asked me about my evening. There was nothing remarkable to report. I had spent my afternoon with him.

Again, I asked, "How are you feeling?"

"Oh, I'm okay," he said. "But my right shoulder hurts."

"Well, I hope you didn't break anything. Can you move it?"

"Yes, but it's sore."

I realized we would have a long wait ahead, as he would obviously need X-rays and CT scans.

Even in these early-morning hours, he seemed as per usual. In these unfamiliar surroundings he was more disoriented. When asked his age, he proudly stated that he was 101 years old. I always found it amazing that the doctors kept asking him the questions, rather than me, when he was not able to answer correctly.

He asked the doctor how long he had worked at the hospital. Eight years, the doctor replied. Dad said, "So you must really find this a good place for you. Do you hope to work in this environment for a while?" The doctor seemed taken aback, surprised to hear Dad's interest. I felt relieved that Dad appeared "normal" after the fall, even if he didn't know his age.

Dad also flirted with the woman taking his blood pressure, checking his temperature, and changing his diaper. When I went to the desk to ask for help, all the nurses remarked that being with my father was very touching.

There was something different about him that night. Maybe it was an extra layer of innocence. He was so dependent, so searching. There was a sense of calm about him. Maybe I just hadn't seen it as clearly before as I did now, in this setting. Or maybe there was something different about him. He appreciated the kindness shown him and returned it in kind. And he stayed awake throughout his stay in the ER.

He accepted that I was there to help him. We talked a bit about how things were going, about Mom, Jan, Craig, and Laurie, and—of course—about the great-grandchildren.

The CT-scan and X-rays came back normal. I drove him back to the memory Unit in time for breakfast. I was exhausted and slept for the rest of the morning.

I returned to him in the afternoon. He had changed. We exchanged hellos, but then he started mumbling. I took him to the nurse, and after a couple of minutes of talking with him, he was better. He seemed as aware as usual and engaged appropriately for him when spoken to. So I hoped that he just needed a good night's sleep. I know that I felt weaker having had little sleep the night before.

The next morning I woke knowing I had to get to the memory unit early to check on him. I found him still having trouble finding words. This time I took him to the nursing supervisor. I knew that I wanted a person in authority to evaluate Dad now. She began to ask him a set of questions, and he said, with a furrowed brow, "can't find words" and mumbled a good deal. He referred back to his mother and father, whom he didn't normally mention. She called the supervising physician saying that Dad had had a change in status after a fall the previous day. She left two messages for the doctor in four minutes. It was urgent. She was concerned. When the doctor returned the call, he sent us back to the ER.

This time the CT scan showed a subdural hematoma, small and inoperable, but it could be treated with plasma and vitamin K. Maybe this wouldn't get any worse. After all, he had a diagnosis of a subdural hematoma before and it had resolved itself.

My mother and brother joined us at the hospital. I had to remind the staff that as a diabetic, Dad needed food. But he was in good spirits, expressing confidence in the people in the hospital working on him. My mother seemed on edge, nervous, and unsure of herself.

Hours later, after completing the meds and promising to return the next day for follow-up examinations, we departed. I went to get my car while two health care workers wheeled my parents to the ambulance bay.

Driving to the entrance to pick them up, seeing them side by side in their wheelchairs, I couldn't help thinking of both of them decades before. I could never keep up with my father when we walked side by side. He kept a fast stride. My mother, too, in her earlier years would walk with great determination. And here they were, the two of them, in wheelchairs and waiting for me in an ambulance bay, toward the end of their lives. I remembered them dancing, being creative, and being a part of life in a very different way.

When we got in the car, Mom, feeling spent, said, "You can take me home first, please."

"Sorry, Mom, I can't leave Dad on his own in the car. I'll take him back and then take you home. And then I'll go back and stay with him."

On the two-mile ride back to the memory unit, Dad remarked, "Hey, you got new tires."

Dad had noticed the week before that the ride in my Honda was uneven and suggested that I needed new tires. I had bought them just two days before.

"Who paid for them?"

"Why, you did, Dad." Even though it wasn't true, I felt that this white lie served a higher good. If this gesture would make him feel better, then it was great.

"Good. Glad it's taken care of." Then his speech turned into mumbling.

It was time to get Mom home. My mother looked anxious. We ate something light, relying on leftovers in the refrigerator. Mom said something about hospice, and I said that we really didn't know if he needed that. What I did know is that I had to return and spend the night there in case he needed anything or there was a problem.

When I got back to the facility, his nurse's aide told me that she had just gotten him ready for bed.

I walked to his room, where I found him on his knees next to his bed.

"Gosh, Dad, did you try to get up and fall?" The aide came in upset.

We got him back in bed. But because of all the IV fluids, he felt the need to urinate at least every hour. And of course he always wanted to go to the bathroom. So instead I convinced him to go in the plastic canister.

At one point he looked at me and asked, "What do women do?"

I just laughed. It was an interesting question at the moment.

For one stretch, he slept in his bed as I slumbered on the lounge chair. He woke suddenly, waking me.

"Oh, Eve, there you are. God sent you to me." He stared not at me, but into the distance. "You know, I've lived a full life. I'm fine."

If nothing else, I knew that despite how confusing his world might appear, when it came to knowing his heart, he was content. I admired him at this moment, once again, for being a brave man.

Chapter 23
Love Watch

We had agreed to return to the hospital the following day to do another CT scan. The subdural hematoma had gotten bigger, but Dad was the same. Would they suggest surgery? During one of those long waiting periods in the ER between doctor visits and test results, as Dad slept, I was feeling burdened by the need to make a decision regarding surgery. I wanted to stay in denial as long as possible that this might be life threatening. I had moved to Florida to help and to be with him. I didn't want him to die. And I certainly didn't want to have to make the decisions about medical procedures. I wanted to just remain in my attachment to him. He was my Dad, the person who had always defined my sense of security. Where would I find that, once he was gone?

In this moment I prayed to let it all go. I did not want to make this decision about his life. It was up to God. In this busy, noisy moment, I laid my forehead on the metal bar around the bed, closed my eyes and hoped that God hangs out in hospital ERs. I prayed to God and all the archangels to take this decision to their realm or to help to find the answers as to what to do for him and what he would want. One moment it seemed so clear what to do, and the next moment fear and doubt clouded my heart and mind. While I was in the midst of my prayers, Dad woke up suddenly. I explained the problem and a possible surgical solution.

He said, "I don't care. I don't care."

I asked him, "What do you mean that you don't care?"

"I'm 91 years old and ahead of the game."

I thanked God for hearing my prayers and having Dad say what at that moment brought clarity for me.

When the neurosurgeon came in, he was presenting the option of surgery to relieve the pressure from the hematoma. Dad spoke to him with clarity and great emphasis, almost to the point of anger, saying: "I'm 91 years old. I've lived my life."

I spoke with the doctor, saying that we would follow Dad's wishes.

In the hallway, the doctor turned to me and said, "You know that we can't rely on his opinion."

I was incredulous. I understood immediately that in the interest of protecting the rights of our elders, we often mistakenly take their rights away. How could one ignore such moments of clarity about the basic decisions in one's life? Are we as a community, and are we as a culture, so confused about what constitutes clarity and understanding? Without Dad's input, I might have gone forward and explored a procedure out of my love, my needs, and my attachment, but I would not have been honoring him.

Over the years, our family had had many conversations about what Dad would want. We all felt comfortable choosing not to take advantage of the treatment. Dad had too many risk factors, and the doctor believed that he wouldn't regain his speech. We had to respect Dad's wishes, even if it meant that he would not live.

I took him back to the memory unit and left briefly to eat. When I came back they told me that he had been unresponsive for a half an hour. He didn't look unhappy, but like he was sleeping too soundly to be awoken. I was totally committed to what I had been hearing Dad say. He was prepared to go. But the aides were shaking him and trying to wake him. They were saying how his roommate was bothering them, something that apparently always managed to produce Dad's ire. I told the nurse we were ready to get hospice care, but I didn't want to move him. Dad woke during the phone conversation. He couldn't speak, but he was awake.

Meanwhile, the nurse had phoned the supervising physician, who said that because Dad had shown a period of unresponsiveness and was not yet enrolled in a hospice program, we would have to go back to the hospital. Even in this wonderful facility, we were trapped in protocols. Dad was sent back to the hospital emergency room, this time in an ambulance.

Again, my brother, mother, and I were on the scene. We made some jokes. Doctors came in, with the same surgical options. Jan and her husband arrived.

Dad could no longer speak, but he was so happy to have us surrounding him. He kept trying to keep track of us, as if he were counting us. He made his opinions known through pantomime, participating in the conversation through elaborate hand motions, and laughing at our jokes. When he spotted my brother-in-law, he called to him, "*shagetz!*" This is the Yiddish word for a non-Jewish man—and it was a joke between my father and Alex, whom my father called "the best *shagetz* in the world." Even if he couldn't form a full sentence, my father's humor and affections were still intact.

Dad was glowing. Even the aide got in the act. As she finished changing him and taking his blood pressure, he took her face in his hands and gave her a long look. He could no longer say thank you. She turned away, crying.

By the next afternoon, he was semi-comatose. He could no longer swallow. We enrolled him into a hospice program. He had only rare moments that he could look at us, and only briefly.

Once, when Jan and I were in the room, the now quite familiar neurosurgeon came in. "What are you doing here?" he asked.

I was a little embarrassed. "Well, doctor, we got lost in the protocols. He was unresponsive at the memory unit, and we didn't yet have him in hospice, so according to their protocols, he had to go to the hospital."

There was now a knowing look on his face about how Dad had wound up on this unit. He helped us to get Dad off medications, and explained that this would probably lead to seizures. He said it could take a week or more before Dad would die.

In my experience as an acupuncturist and energy worker, I had decades of experience working with people at the end of their lives. Often, they were dying of cancer. Once I overheard someone I didn't know very well referring to me as a hospice healer. I looked at this time in a person's life as similar to a birth process, where you go through many ups and downs, and there is a sense of waiting for a big event.

I always found that the time before their death seemed long—it has an endless quality. I wanted us to live a love watch, rather than a death-watch. I wanted the love to seem endless, not the stress. I was committed to have his remaining time be loving and calm. I wanted him to never be alone. I wanted to make sure that there was the fine quality to his death that there had been to his life. And I had promised him many times over the past two years that I would make sure he was able to die well.

The memory unit enrolled him in their hospice program, and it seemed only fitting that we continue to use their help. I had no idea what a great decision it would be to be there. It was wonderful to have the help of people who had known Dad over the past year, people who had genuine affection for him.

With the arrival of Jan and Alex, our family took up every bed and couch in Craig and Mom's apartment. There was not enough room to also make Dad comfortable at their home. With staff shortages during the Christmas holidays, Jan, Craig and I had to cover some of the shifts at the memory unit. We were constantly tending Dad.

I spent the night in Dad's room his first night back from the hospital. At 3:30 a.m. he started having seizures. I had seen grand mal seizures before. But in this situation it wasn't one seizure and then a return to normal. Dad was totally out of it, asleep, and semi-comatose. He would wake to a seizure, then five minutes later, have another. I would press on acupuncture points and tell him to breathe with me, which he would do. I assured him that we would take care of him and he wouldn't be suffering. When he was awake and alert, I would explain his situation, saying that he was in hospice and he would be cared for, and we would get the situation with the seizures under control. There was no doubt in my mind that he understood every word I said.

While the nurse was helping to get meds, transitioning us out of one program and into another, I was feeling frazzled and exhausted. I was turning into one long contracted muscle. Dad must have had at least a dozen seizures in a two-hour time period. By the morning, I was at my breaking point. I pulled the alarm to get the nurse and four of the nurses' aides came running in. They stood shocked and frozen at finding Dad having a seizure.

I reassured them that all was well, but that I wanted the nurse to see if she knew anything more to do before we could get him medicated. She stayed with us the next half-hour tending to his immediate problems.

Now that he was having seizures, he was eligible for 24-hour nursing care through hospice. Thank God for the goodness of hospice to provide so much comfort as people move into transition from this life.

Quickly we figured out a schedule where a family member could be there most hours of the day and night. We took care of Dad's needs, moistening his lips, checking whether he seemed to be in any pain, cleaning him, and turning him every two hours. I made an essential oil blend which we used to massage his hands. Jan and I sang to him.

◇

On one of my shifts I went to the dining area looking for Dad's nursing aide to help me to turn him. One of the aides, who I was sure wasn't Dad's aide, asked me what I needed.

At the moment she seemed quite busy, but she volunteered to help me. Her face was familiar, and she wore a large jeweled cross.

"I'm so sorry," I said. "I've seen you and spoken with you before, but I can't remember your name."

"Barbara," she said.

I started laughing. "Barbara! I have heard quite a bit about you." Everyone working there knew that Dad loved Barbara and wanted her to marry him. He talked about how he was facing a big obstacle, in that she was already married. He lamented his bad luck.

"Barbara, do you want to know what Dad said to me about you?"

"What?" she asked, giggling a little.

"He said, 'She's as beautiful on the inside as she is on the outside.'"

She held herself back from crying, and looked down for a moment, composing herself.

I said, "You know, he really saw you."

We went in and gently moved Dad from his left side to his right, placing pillows carefully to prevent skin breakage. I was still tentative in moving Dad in his increasingly fragile state. How different this was from when I arrived just over a month before. I had thought then that I would get to enjoy being with Dad for six months or more.

I was glad to give his Barbara the benefit of our private father/daughter conversations. Recognizing another human being's loving heart is always significant.

◇

We contended with obstacles in getting Dad 24-hour nursing care during the Christmas holidays. Sometimes the hospice nurse didn't show up for her shift, and I would get a call at 2 a.m., saying there was no nurse. I went to the facility and waited until my sister could take the next shift.

On one of those long nights, a lovely aide named Anna helped me. She told me she was originally from Honduras. We started talking about dementia, and she told me the story of her grandfather, who had been living with their family in New York City. He woke up once in the middle of the night with only his underwear on and went wandering through the neighborhood.

When Anna and her family woke, they searched for her grandfather, finally finding him at the police station, just as happy as could be. Their solution was to have him return to Honduras, where he could live in a small village where people had known him for decades. These people returned him home if he wandered.

It seemed so sane, to return home to the places where people know you and will take care of your needs, showing you directions, just as you used to show them.

As she told me the story, I hoped that Dad, now semi-comatose, could still feel his way and find the familiar way home.

One afternoon as my niece visited, Dad came out of his semi-comatose state. Laurie showed him pictures of the great-grandchildren, and he couldn't take his eyes off of them. Because he seemed frustrated not being able to talk, she told him that there was nothing that he had not already said to her, and she knew how much he loved her.

She was saying her goodbyes to him, as it was time to pick up her children. He grasped her hand. He didn't want her to leave.

She called us to come, as he was awake and holding on. We all arrived quickly—Jan, Alex, Craig, Mom, and I. I watched my father have his moment of attachment and love for his granddaughter. He did not have eyes for another person. Even though he couldn't speak, his eyes spoke his love and his expression echoed the one that I had seen just two weeks before, at the Chanukah party, when he said, "I miss everyone." Now he was in the reality of his heart, knowing that he would always miss his granddaughter.

This was the last time he looked at any of us. He floated into a semi-comatose state. The nurses touched his face to see whether he was responsive or not. In those last days of his life, we stayed with him, talking with him, telling him we loved him and that we cared for his needs in our love watch.

On December 27, 2004, Laurie, Jan, Alex, Craig, and I spent the morning visiting with him, telling our individual stories of Dad, and talking about the future of the great-grandchildren. We all left to have lunch. He died during that hour.

I laughed that Dad would never have left us if we were in the room. He would be too interested in what we were saying. But I knew that he had died just the way that I had promised him: beautifully, peacefully, and perfectly.

Epilogue

I moved home to Florida for what I thought would be the whole winter, but within a month of my arrival, Dad had passed. After the ordeal of it all, I needed rest and to collect myself. And I was numb. I recall how one day soon after the funeral, Craig, Jan, and I just sat on the couch too exhausted to do more than say a few words to each other. We each ached in our own way from the loss.

I was living with Mom and Craig, taking occasional teaching gigs in Miami or Tucson, but finding that I was the odd person out in Orlando. My lifestyle and habits were too different from theirs. I wasn't being very helpful to Craig. The incompatibility outweighed the urge to help. So I left to pursue my own dreams, ambitions, and joy.

As a child, my grandparents had lived in Phoenix, and Arizona was always on my short list of places I wanted to live because of my early memories of that vast landscape. I moved to Tucson, where I easily developed a practice, made friendships, and took daily hikes into the mountains. I had possibilities again.

About two years after Dad's death, Craig called me crying. I'd never heard him cry before. He called saying he had stage 3 non-large-cell lung cancer. It was as if a bomb went off in my life. Everything went on pause. My practice. My new life in Tucson. This book.

I had many years of experience working with cancer patients, and I understood immediately that I would most likely lose my brother. I was in shock but determined to support him through any treatment. I immediately sought out a therapist to help me handle the grief and anger at the prospect of losing my amazing brother, but much of the time I still talked of my father and where I was in my loss around his death.

When I visited Craig, I treated him with acupuncture three times a day. Craig had the best attitude. We spent much of the time laughing. I asked him if he could have anything in the world now what would it be. And he answered, "Meg Ryan." So I tried contacting her for an autographed picture or some memento. I couldn't get through to her, but one day, I told him the story of my pursuit. He was surprised, and hung on every word. Then he laughed and joked about what a disappointment it was that she didn't answer.

Craig did much better than the physicians at MD Anderson Clinic in Orlando thought possible, with his primary tumor shrinking. I would have the gift of more time with him.

I left Tucson and moved to Maryland to be close to my sister. If and when Craig passed, my sister, brother-in-law, and I would be responsible for my mother. To nourish my spirit, I pursued my Chinese Medicine studies.

Craig passed in April 2009. His lightness of spirit is something I will always treasure and miss.

Jan and I brought Mom up to Maryland. She quickly forgot that my brother had died. When she initially asked where he was, I mistakenly answered that he had passed, being astonished that she didn't remember his funeral. That first time I told her she cried and asked me when were we planning to tell her. Within another half hour, she asked me again. I never made that same mistake. I always said he was busy and couldn't get to her this week. Our worlds no longer matched. We no longer even shared this pain.

However, Mom took great pleasure in some parts of her journey. In her memory unit, they had musical programs most days. Mom always had an amazing musical talent. That was true even in her last years. When she was living in the memory unit, she really thought that everyone was there to see her perform. This was a highlight of her time. She had COPD and congestive heart failure and was on oxygen 24/7, but she could still belt out a song like she was on stage. In a strange way, she was happy and fulfilled.

During many of the visits over the next four years, Mom just yelled at me. It was a shock to have her stuck in this anger. Her ways of interacting changed entirely. Sometimes I couldn't make sense out of her sentences. Sometimes she yelled in Yiddish. It was clear from her expression that she didn't know why I couldn't understand her.

Jan and I had known it would be challenging to care for her. This was not surprising. But I had no idea that she would be so abusive. During the abusive outbursts, Jan simply walked out, telling Mom that she would see her later in the week. I felt like I should be able to help get her back to some calmer part of herself, like we often were able to do with Dad, but nothing worked. I would leave and need to purge the entire experience out of my psyche and body.

One night at least two years into caring for Mom, I thought I was finished. I couldn't take any more of this abuse. In fact, my mother herself, in her healthy days, wouldn't have approved of maintaining such an abusive relationship. After I went to bed crying, I had a one-on-one with God. I said I would rather die than put myself in an ongoing abusive situation, even with my mother. I was ready to die or God could take her, but I was not going to keep going if this didn't change. I felt like I was shirking my responsibility. I didn't know how this might play out, but I was sure that I needed to take some radical action.

With my next visit, the abuse stopped. While I was really talking with the Divine, something had finally shifted in her. She was calmer and stopped being in attack mode. We were able to proceed with a greater amount of love and respect between us.

Sometimes she had brief moments as her old self. She turned to me once and said, "Evie, there's something wrong with the way I'm thinking. What's wrong with me?" As I was trying to formulate a way to explain it to her, she started to go back to being confused.

Caring for my mom was a different experience than caring for my dad. I am like my father in some ways—amiable, interested in people, fair, curious. But I am also relentless, compassionate, creative, and spiritual, like my mother. While we mirror for each other, I've also learned that we can acknowledge our own gifts.

Through these experiences, I have a way of appreciating my own gifts now that I might have overlooked or discounted before. In almost every letter Dad wrote he urged us to "live a good life." Using my gifts and sharing them with the world will always be my way of living a good life.

As I accompanied my father and later my mother on the journey with dementia, I gained a deeper personal revelation about the basic dignity in every moment of a person's life. Honoring these moments is seen as a challenge when the person changes. It is demanding in ways I would know only through having the experience. It's demanding to function when you are rarely in the same reality. But it is truly demanding to value the difference, as if you are exploring knowing this person for the first time. Even without history and memories, you still have something more basic that you share: Love.

Acknowledgments

I would not have attempted to write this book without the support and encouragement of my brother, sister, niece, and mother. I love you all.

My friend Dirk Walters helped me through the emotional trials as well as the difficulties in putting the words on the page. He always said that it could be done, when I was sure that it couldn't.

And to my myriad friends who through thick and thin listened to these stories with compassionate ears and allowed my heartaches to reach them, I bow. So thank you Sue Greer for your wisdom, Ruth Pettus for your timely calls, Kate McGee for your generosity, Shoshana Kornan for the walks around the lake, Guiliana Reed for your compassion, Elizabeth Finley for your ability to assess reality, Mimi Ratner for your sensitivity, Suzy Murphy for your knowledge, Susan Klein for endless sympathy, Denyce Graves for your heart, Connie McKenna for reading the early drafts, Jan Carpenter for your willingness to come and hold my hand, Komala Lyra for being my inspiration, Warren Bellows for reminding me of my inner core, Ann

Bailey for your sensitivity, Judith Brown for cheering me forward, Sandy and Michael Morse for endless support, and Sandy Camper for always being willing to laugh with me. Many thanks to everyone at Circle Center in Fairfax, California, for being a part of my spiritual family during this entire time.

And a special thank you to my cousin Elaine Soldinger, who kept up with the ups and downs the entire time.

Thank you, Esther Goldenberg of Three Gems Publishing, who after I had spent years thinking that I would never finish this book helped me discover that it was already finished. Thank you for helping me to push along this process.

Thank you to my editors Mary Smith, Sara Wildberger, and Derry Koralek for your contributions in making this a beautiful read.

ABOUT THE AUTHOR

Eve Soldinger, MPH, M.Ac., MMQ, Dipl.Ac.(NCCAOM), has always studied and taught about transformation and spiritual healing. She has traveled widely to study with indigenous men and women, expert healers, and profound practitioners of Chinese medical knowledge, and she finds that our deepest healing comes through nature. Eve found everything that she studied and sought to discover had to be called upon to be present in this challenging situation with her parents. It was a difficult but meaningful journey, and she hopes that this story gives you support on whatever your journey presents.

Eve lives in Silver Spring, MD and enjoys the preciousness of life, and is always grateful to be a practitioner of Chinese Medicine. She can be reached at www.EveSoldinger.com.

Made in the USA
Middletown, DE
18 March 2016